Recently published in Corgi Mini-Books

BARBARA CARTLAND

THE YOUTH SECRET

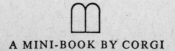

A MINI-BOOK BY CORGI

THE YOUTH SECRET

A MINI-BOOK 552 06098 4
PRINTING HISTORY
Mini-Book Edition published 1968
Reprinted 1968
Reprinted 1968
Reprinted 1969
Reprinted 1970
Reprinted 1971
Mini-Books are published by Transworld Publishers Ltd.,
Cavendish House, 57–59 Uxbridge Road, Ealing,
London, W.5
Made and Printed in Great Britain by
Fletcher & Son Ltd., Norwich

Contents

CHAPTER I

Stay Young

'Hell, I look a million!' said Tana, turning a desperate face towards the mirror on her dressing-table.

'Nonsense!' I replied. 'I think you look charming.'

'Do you realise,' she asked, turning round to face me, 'that I shall be fifty tomorrow? Fifty! I used to think everyone of that age ought to be exterminated, they were so old!'

'We don't think things like that today,' I said. 'Women are charming, clever, beautiful and successful until they are really very old in years, but even so they can still seem young. And, what is far more important, feel young.'

'You must tell me how,' Tana said, 'because when I reached my fortieth birthday I really didn't feel any different. But I do think fifty is a tremendous milestone. After all it's half a century!'

'Stop thinking about it like that,' I said. 'Think as it as only half your age. Scientists are already telling us we shall live to be a hundred!'

'And who wants to live to be a hundred?' Tana asked. 'Old, wrinkled, rheumatic and not capable of enjoying anything.'

'That is the whole point,' I said quietly. 'We all want to live young. We want to feel young; we want to be able to do all the things that we could do when we were young and however old we may be in years, I believe it is possible we can do just that.'

'How?' Tana asked. 'Just tell me how, that's what I want.'

'Well, I will try,' I replied. 'First of all, I want to fill you in with the background as to why people today feel ill, worried and jittery; why so many are having psychiatric treatment; or, worse still, why millions spend some part of their life in a mental home.'

'You know the answer?' Tana enquired, wide-eyed.

'I do, indeed,' I replied. 'The answer is – you are what you eat.'

'Oh, that's an old story!' she said petulantly, obviously disappointed at my reply.

'Unfortunately it is true,' I said. 'You see, what people never realise is that every day they are building up or destroying part of their health. If you were an athlete you wouldn't expect to eat all sorts of fattening foods, drink a lot of alcohol, smoke and stay up to the early hours of the morning before you ran a big race. You would know that you would be beaten from the start. But that is exactly what ordinary people are doing and they are being beaten by their opponent – Old Age – when they are still very young!'

'Go on,' Tana encouraged me.

I could see she was interested.

'You have to look on old age as 'the enemy',' I said. 'We've all read about the elixir of youth which was sought by famous alchemists and a great many crooks in the Middle Ages. They concocted potions which people drank, rubbed on themselves, slept with under their pillows and imagined the magic would work. The

extraordinary thing is that only a few people ever
realised where the real secret lay. One of these was
Diane de Poitiers. She refused to indulge in the rich,
exotic foods that were served in the King's palace and,
instead, exercised every day, bathed in cold water and
ate a diet of fruit and vegetables combined with what
her enemies thought was a concoction of the devil.'

'What was it?' Tana asked.

'It was a soup made from venison, hares, pheasants,
and partridges,' I said. 'Now you realise what that soup
was, don't you? It was protein! That is why Diane
remained supremely beautiful until she died. The King
of France, Henry II, eighteen years her junior, was
passionately in love with her until he was killed in a
joust; she was then sixty. Very old in the terms of the
Middle Ages.'

'Well, do I go out and catch a hare and make a soup?'
Tana laughed.

'Unfortunately, today it is far more difficult than it
was in Diane's day,' I replied. 'You see, owing to the
craziness of mankind, we are doing our best to destroy
ourselves. We pour aerosols, pesticides and chemicals
of all types into the soil until it is polluted.'

'I have read 'Silent Spring' as it happens,' Tana interposed.

'So have most sensible people,' I said, 'because it is the
most terrifying warning of what can happen in a civilised country. But having poisoned the soil, the chemicals have seeped into the streams and rivers and
combined with the toxic waste that comes from our
factories, it has proceeded into the sea so that we have

9

now polluted the sea seventy miles out.'

'It can't be true!' Tana exclaimed.

'Unfortunately, it is,' I said. 'Every fish that is caught round the shores of Great Britain, and the same applies to the United States, contains pesticides. They are even picking up seagulls' eggs in Iceland with D.D.T. in them.'

'I thought D.D.T. was no longer allowed to be used,' Tana said.

'So do most people,' I replied. 'Unfortunately, statistics show us that over 500,000 tons was used in Great Britain last year and a great deal more in some other countries. It is now estimated that every human being and animal in all civilised countries now has a D.D.T. build-up in their body fat.'

'It sounds terrifying!' Tana cried.

'It is terrifying,' I replied. 'And when you think that farmers give tranquilisers to beef cattle and to pigs so that they fatten quicker; when you think they caponise chickens with stilboestrol, which is a female hormone which is a proven cancer inducer in rats; that our eggs come from batteries and all our vegetables are sprayed; are you surprised that we are worried at the toxic condition of the human race.'

'It is crazy,' Tana murmured.

'Besides all this,' I went on, '2,000 chemicals are used in our food. These preserve, colour, flavour, harden, soften, liquify, emulsify, thicken or thin but not one of them has any nutritive value! The Food and Drugs Commissioner in the United States has said about these chemicals: 'Some of them are so poisonous they will kill human beings instantly if eaten in large doses, but industrial chemists have argued they are safe because they are consumed in small amounts – an argument which is the heart of the problem'.'

'It doesn't seem possible,' Tana ejaculated.

'Unfortunately, it is not only possible but is something which is actually happening,' I replied. 'And this is where we begin to see old age and perhaps death creeping ahead of us and destroying us almost before we have begun to enjoy this very wonderful life of ours.'

'One of the things which I am convinced comes from this over-consumption of toxic chemicals is the increase of cancer. Professor A. Berglas of the L'Institut Pasteur in Paris has said that if we go on as we are adding toxic chemicals to the air we breathe, the water we drink and to every particle of our food, before very long everybody will be threatened with death through cancer.'

Tana shuddered.

'Cancer is the one thing that frightens me.'

'We all are,' I replied. 'And the cancer figures are appalling. More than one in six in this country die of cancer – one in four in the U.S.A. – and more children under twelve die of cancer than are killed on the road!'

'Children too!' Tana said. 'Surely we shall soon find a cure.'

'I would prefer to prevent this horrible disease,' I replied. 'We know that where there is no civilization there is no cancer – for example the Hunzas and Ethiopians. Where civilization starts to change the nutrition, cancer develops. But for all of us there is tremendous hope in the fact that it has been discovered that cancer

11

can be prevented by eating the right food or, rather, by consuming the right amount of vitamins.'

'But how can we be certain that our food contains the right amount of vitamins?' Tana asked.

'That is a very clever question,' I told her, 'and one I hoped you would ask. Because, you see, we can't. As I've already said, man has destroyed the soil, the sea, polluted the air and practically every foodstuff we touch has in some way been treated by chemicals. Therefore, there is only one thing we can do.'

'And what is that?' Tana asked eagerly.

'It sounds rather Alice in Wonderland,' I answered. 'But we must put back into our bodies what ought to be on our plates.'

'And this will make all the difference?' Tana enquired.

'It will indeed,' I answered. 'In an experiment in America they gave rats Butter Yellow, which was a very dangerous dye used for a great number of years, I regret to say, in the colouring of butter until it was found to cause cancer of the liver. The rats taking Butter Yellow developed liver cancer in 150 days, which is a very short time. The rats were then given Butter Yellow plus 15 per cent Brewers' Yeast. Not one single rat developed cancer! Similar experiments have taken place with Vitamin A and guinea pigs. Now that is, to me, a conclusive proof that though the dangers are all around us we can combat them with the antedote of the right and correct food.'

'Perhaps we could just eat vitamins alone?' Tana suggested brightly.

'That is an idea which many people have had,' I said,

'but it doesn't work. You have got to have food plus vitamins.'

'I've often heard doctors say that we get all the vitamins that we need in our food,' Tana said.

'I'm afraid they are old-fashioned and out-of-date,' I replied. 'My answer to that is very simple. Most people have no idea what they are eating. For instance, a short time ago the Birmingham City Analyst took samples of nine foods which were being consumed in the City. Five of them, he discovered, contained non-permitted dyes which had been banned in this country for years! We are never certain when these dangerous substances will be discovered and how many are being used of which we know nothing.'

'What should we avoid?' Tana enquired.

'I wish I could answer that,' I replied. 'I keep thinking of a noted cancer researcher who said, 'The growing custom of introducing an endless series of biologically foreign molecules into the human organism is not unlike throwing a collection of nuts and bolts into the most delicate machinery known.''

'Surely we can learn which 'nuts and bolts' to avoid?' Tana asked.

'The danger of consuming toxic chemicals,' I replied, 'is that taken in small amounts they work slowly to bring sickness and death, but they often appear quite harmless. Take Dulcin, for instance, Dulcin is an artificial sweetening agent. It was used for more than half a century as a substitute for sugar by manufacturers before it was found to sause cancer in animals. Another ingredient, Coumarin, an imitation vanilla flavour, was used

13

for 75 years in a wide variety of confectionery before it was discovered to produce serious liver damage in animals.'

'I suppose no-one uses them now?' Tana said.

'There are others,' I replied. 'Take another flavour – pineapple; it usually comes from ethyl acetate, which is better known as a solvent for plastics and lacquers. Its vapour is well-known to be irritating to the mucous membranes and if you are exposed to it for some time it can cause chronic pulmonary, liver and heart damage.'

'I shall never buy anything that says it is flavoured with pineapple again!' Tana exclaimed.

'It's very difficult to avoid these things,' I replied. 'Look at cheese. Processed cheese is little more than a complex of chemicals. It is artificially thickened, stabilised, preserved, flavoured and coloured. One of the thickeners used in processed cheese is called methyl cellulose. This is also used to make cosmetic and adhesives. And another stabiliser sodium carboxymethyl is used in resin-emulsion paints and printing inks. Even a cheese wrapper is treated with chemicals. Recently, 60,000 pounds of these was seized because the chemicals used in the wrapping had seeped into the cheese. It was quite tasteless and completely odourless and yet it was as poisonous as carbolic acid.'

'You're terrifying me!' Tana said.

'Let me tell you another frightening thing,' I went on. 'To prevent the spoilage of carrots, oranges, apples, lemons and limes they have now invented a wax which is made of a coal-tar-derivitive paraffin which is highly suspect as a cause of cancer. What is so disgraceful is

14

that the chemicals we use in food are accepted if they qualify for the technical job demanded of them and no further questions are asked. All that their manufacturers require is that they shall make money. Will they keep a cake from falling? Will they quickly and cheaply add to the weight of meat animals? Will they firm tomatoes and stiffen pickles? Will they keep the mould off bread? Will they tenderise the steak and give it a certain flavour? If the chemical is able to perform its job without immediately killing a test animal, then why should the consumer complain?'

'But, what can we do about it?' Tana asked.

'Well, you can first start to understand what is happening in the world around you,' I said. 'You've said you want to remain young and beautiful. Look at it from a purely selfish point of view. Unless you can preserve your body, your skin and your brain from all these dangers, then you are gradually going to lose the one thing you want to keep – your youth.'

'Tell me more,' Tana begged.

'I will,' I answered. 'But I want you to realise that this is something that most people laugh at or else ignore because they just don't want to know. People wish to live their lives easily and comfortably. It's a bore to have to fuss about the food that comes to the table. It's extra trouble to seek out Health Stores, to find farmers who will sell free-range eggs or gardeners who grow organic vegetables. It's also expensive to buy natural vitamins – those same vitamins that ought to be on your plate but which aren't.'

'Why can't we get them on the National Health?' Tana

asked.

'Because,' I replied, 'they are a food; definitely a food and not a medicine. The vitamins that a doctor can give you on a prescription are all synthetic. They are made in factories from chemicals and therefore you are only adding to the toxic condition of your body when you take them.'

'And you really think the taking of vitamins makes a difference to our health?' Tana asked.

'I can only tell you about my Mother,' I said. 'Of course, she didn't begin to take vitamins until about ten years ago. But she's now over ninety. She drives her own car everywhere and cleans it! She has more energy than most young women. She is on a dozen committees. She has fetes, 'Bring and Buy' sales and committee meetings at her house incessantly. She speaks on 'Looking back 90 years' and she says, quite openly and frankly, that if it wasn't for vitamins she wouldn't be able to do any of these. In fact, she might easily be dead.'

'Well, that certainly is a recommendation!' Tana exclaimed.

'I only wish that I could have started to take vitamins earlier in my life,' I said. 'I believe that those little wrinkles I see coming around my eyes and round my mouth would not be there and I'm quite certain that instead of writing 115 books by now, I would have written 315.'

'If it's going to make me work hard,' Tana teased, 'I don't think I want to hear any more.'

'You'll work because you enjoy working,' I said. 'You'll find that you have a new zest in life, a new interest in everything you do. The sad thing is that at least three quarters of the people in this country are not really well. In fact we are a Sick Nation, with 300 million working days lost last year through illness. People drag themselves along, they muddle through, but they feel tired and irritable, limp and often mentally exhausted. And it's all so unnecessary!'

'Do you feel well?' Tana asked.

'I resent it if I don't feel 100 per cent every day of my life,' I answered.

'Well, make me feel like that,' Tana said, 'because I not only feel and look tired, but I am extremely irritable.'

'Then let us start right away,' I said. 'Let us take the first step towards the exciting exploration of eternal youth!'

CHAPTER II

The Brain

'What do we start with?' Tana asked. 'My body?'

'I think if I was asked what was the most important part of a person,' I answered, 'I would say the brain. What people never seem to realise is that food actively affects the brain. The Salvation Army produced a report on delinquents in which they proved that both boys and girls who were difficult, hard to get on with, obstreperous and even young toughs who hit people over the head with a bicycle chain, could become quite normal when properly fed.'

'I would like to read that,' Tana said.

'It was really a sensational report which was brought out some six or seven years ago,' I said. 'It didn't attract very much attention because people, as a general rule, just don't believe it. And then in 1964 Dr. Richard MacKarness told the International Congress of Social Psychiatry in London a most fascinating story. He said that a mother who found her seven year old child beyond her control brought the litte boy to see him. Michael was a terror! He smashed his toys, hit his brothers and was so unmanageable that no-one could do anything with him. He stammered, bit his nails, suffered from insomnia and could not concentrate at school.'

'Dr. MacKarness found out that the things Michael liked eating best were iced lollies and cornflakes – of course, covered with white sugar. Dr. MacKarness persuaded the mother to eliminate from Michael's diet all processed foods and food of cereal origin. To everyone's astonishment, at the end of the week Michael was behaving like a normal child. He was happy, good-tempered, easy to live with and obedient.'

'Dr. MacKarness told the Conference that the mother was worried that the improvement might be just a coincidence.'

''I persuaded her to re-introduce quite a number of Michael's processed, carbohydrate foods,' he said. 'Cornflakes, white bread, iced lollies, biscuits, cakes and milk chocolate. Within three days he was as irritable as to be almost out of control. But when Michael was put back on his diet he became well again within a few days!''

'What an extraordinary story,' Tana said.

'You do see that this shows a direct relationship between the stomach and the brain?' I asked. 'I often wonder how many marriages crash simply and solely because 'the incompatibility' which takes them to the Courts really originated in the kitchen.'

Tana looked guilty.

'I'm beginning to worry as to whether I feed my husband the right way,' she said. 'I've always thought it was such a bother to make John eggs and bacon before he goes off to the City in the morning. He eats Cornflakes, I think.'

'If you believe those wicked advertisements on the television,' I said, 'that a cereal breakfast is enough for a grown man or for growing children, you'll believe any-

19

thing. We all need protein for breakfest and that is what I am going to order for you.'

'Oh, I can't eat anything,' Tana replied. 'A cup of black coffee is all ever need.'

'You're crazy!' I said sternly. 'Do you realise that when you've fasted for twelve hours, which everyone does at night, the most important meal of the day is breakfast – and the most rejuvenating one?'

'You mean without breakfast I look older?' Tana asked.

'Definitely older,' I answered. 'I can prove it to you. You see, we all have in our bodies something called blood sugar. It has nothing to do with ordinary sugar; it is what gives us energy and keeps us full of vitality and good health. During the night, when you are asleep, your blood sugar drops and in the morning it has to be raised from approximately, we'll say, 64 degrees to 100 degrees. Now, what raises it properly is protein. A cup of coffee will raise it temporarily for a very, very short time and then it drops lower than it was before. Haven't you often found that you're very tired by mid-morning?'

'Of course, I always am,' Tana answered. 'So, then I have another cup of coffee.'

'And you age a great deal at the same time,' I answered.

'I had no idea it was wrong.' Tana exclaimed.

'Most people haven't. And most people have the ridiculous idea that it slims them to cut out breakfast,' I replied. 'They like lunch and they like dinner so they think they'll dispense with breakfast when they don't feel well in the morning. But the reason they don't feel well is because they are eating the wrong things. I wake up in the morning feeling wonderful, and I have for breakfast two eggs, honey and fruit.'

'Every morning?' Tana asked.

'Every morning,' I said. 'Two eggs boiled or poached, a spoonful or two of honey and an apple, or, perhaps, melon in the summertime. And, then of course, I take my vitamins; so I'm ready for a heavy day's work. I don't need 'elevenses'. I never have them.'

'And what do you suggest my John should have?' Tana enquired.

'John should have at least two eggs, bacon and sausages, or ham, brawn or tongue before he goes to the City. Dieticians, like Lelord Kordel eat a steak or several lamb chops. Adelle Davis eats $\frac{1}{2}$-lb. of liver. No bread – that's unnecessary and John doesn't need it; a cup of weak tea and, if he has time, an apple. He'll feel well and he'll get through the day far better and with far less exhaustion than if he'd gulped down a few spoonsful of sugary cereal, or, like you, grabbed a cup of coffee.'

Tana made a grimace.

'I believe that men and women who work are definitely cheating their employers if they don't eat a proper breakfast,' I continued. 'A recent survey showed that men and women were at their mental and physical best an hour after a meal. I look forward to the day when all industrial firms have the commonsense to insist that every employee, when he arrives at work, goes straight to the canteen and has a proper breakfast.'

'You won't get agreement to that,' Tana said.

'Why not?' I enquired. 'It would mean that productivity would go up, I should think, ten to twenty per cent in

21

almost every firm. And instead of seeing shop girls with thin, emaciated figures and white faces, drooping over counters, there would be bright, cheerful young ladies anxious to serve and send away satisfied customers.'

'It sounds wonderful from the customers' point of view,' Tana said. 'But who is going to believe you?'

'I don't think people study the medical reports half as seriously as they should do,' I said. 'Dr. Geoffrey Taylor, two years ago, with a team of researches investigated the problem of old people in a hospital of 500 beds. He went so far as to say that 90 per cent of all old people were suffering from vitamin deficiency and large numbers of them were actually dying from scurvy – lack of vitamin C, which is something we all thought went out with Nelson.'

'But, surely the old people were having milk?' Tana said. 'I thought we got vitamin C in milk?'

'If they were, it wasn't enough,' I answered. 'But personally, I am against milk for adults. So I beg all people who are grown up not to have milk. I think it is something we do not need. Milk was never meant for adults. Nature intended milk for a young animal when it took no other food, and I find that half the young people who have acne, and older people who have migraine, can be cured if they give up milk. Another large group of people in this country suffer from sinusitis and catarrh. Take them off milk and soggy white bread and in 90 per cent of the cases the sinus trouble and the catarrh clears up almost at once.'

'I wish I had known this last winter,' Tana said. 'What a lot there is to learn.'

'I want you to understand the dangers,' I said, 'because unless you understand exactly what you are up against, you are never going to begin to realise how much you have got to help yourself. Nobody else will help you. In this age, it is a terrifying thing that a human baby may begin to absorb toxic chemicals from the moment it begins to feed at its mother's breast. This was proved by the figures in an American study which showed the average of 13 parts of D.D.T. per 100 million in the milk of a group of wet nurses in a hospital.'

'Don't frighten me any more!' Tana begged. 'No milk! And what else mustn't I have?'

'There's a whole list, I'm afraid,' I answered. 'Processed foods; things like white flour – which has been refined until all the goodness has gone out of it; all those gooey, shop-made cakes; most of the things which come in lovely, coloured packets, easy to prepare. They have no value except to destroy your complexion and irritate the stomach.'

'All out!' Tana agreed.

'And while we are still talking about the brain,' I continued, 'you will remember that I started telling you about Michael whose brain was affected by ice-lollies. Now the reason was that ice-lollies, like most of the things that are sold in confectioners, contain white sugar. And white sugar is the most dangerous thing of all!'

'One of our great nutritists called white sugar 'the curse of civilisation'. Scientists are becoming more and more convinced that it is white sugar which is the cause of coronary thrombosis. What we do know is that white

23

sugar steals the vitamins from your body.'

'Explain,' Tana commanded.

'I'm just going to,' I answered. 'And as simply as possible. All the food we eat is alive; it has some life in it – with the exception of white sugar. White sugar has been refined and refined and refined until, to please the silly housewife, all the goodness has gone from it. You know the colour of sugar? I've seen it in Mexico in the sugar cane; I've seen it in Jamaica. It's a dark, thick brown syrup. But when it has gone through all the ridiculous processes to which mankind subjects it, all the vitamins are washed away and there is nothing left except a dead substance which has a special sweet taste. You put it into your live body and your body, because it works that way, says, 'this has got to be digested'. So, it takes vitamins from your heart, vitamins from your kidneys and vitamins from your liver – all vital spots – to get rid of this ghastly, white mess that you have put into your digestive tract.'

'I can understand that,' Tana said. 'No white sugar!'

'Now, to get back to your brain,' I said, 'this dangerous assault on your digestive organs makes you tired and nervous; it gives you headaches and migraine. Just look at the citizens of this country. We are a nation of sufferers from nerves, digestive disorders, tiredness, poor eyesight, anaemia, heart trouble, muscular diseases and hundreds of assorted skin troubles. And I am convinced that a great deal of this suffering is due to the lack of the B vitamins caused by the amount of sugar we eat every year. Give up sugar and you will find that your brain is clearer, you look much more attractive, you feel lighter, gayer, and you automatically become thinner.'

'A most important point,' Tana smiled.

'Just as that child, Michael, was irritated to the point when he could not control his temper,' I continued, ignoring her interruption, 'this happens to adult people in a smaller or greater degree. Take away sugar and people who are extremely bad tempered will often become charming, good tempered and easy to live with. And yet visit any home, however poor, and you see great bowls of white sugar on the table. They will go without meat, they will go without fruit, they will go without anything that does them good, rather than give up white sugar which is, in some ways, a drug!'

'A drug?' Tana ejaculated.

'The workers in sugar factories often put six or more spoonsful of sugar in their tea,' I answered. 'The more they eat the more they want and it goes on destroying the live vitamins in their bodies until their mind becomes affected.'

'But I thought everyone needed something sweet,' Tana said. 'Especially old people.'

'So we do,' I replied. 'And what we should eat is the most wonderful food in the world and also the food of love.'

'I wondered how long we were going to be before we got to love,' Tana said.

'Well, it's starting right now,' I answered. 'Love is something which makes you beautiful, fitter and more effectual as a person than anything else in the whole world. And the food of love is – Honey!'

25

'Is that why we talk about a Honeymoon?' Tana asked.

'The name came from some love cakes given to every Roman bride and bridegroom,' I answered. 'Honey has been used as an aphrodisiac in every country in the world which has a history of medicine. It is also a healer, a strengthener, an energiser and a natural sedative.'

'The last two sound contradictiory,' Tana interposed.

'That is one of the magical qualities of honey,' I replied. 'When the ancient Phoenician traders came to Britain in search of lead and tar they found such enormous quantities of honey that they called it 'the Isle of Honey'. And when Plutarch landed in Britain he was astonished at the health of its people. 'These Britons,' he wrote, 'only begin to grow old at 130 years of life.''

'It makes you live longer!' Tana exclaimed.

'The ancient peoples knew it did,' I answered. 'In those days, honey was the only sweetener in the world. The Greeks at the Olympic Games and those who fought great battles, all knew that honey strengthened and invigorated them.'

'Then why did they change to sugar?' Tana asked.

'It was not until the Middle Ages,' I replied, 'that the very rich started to use sugar, which was called 'honey honey reed'. It was, of course, a snob food and to 'keep up with the Joneses' you had to have it. Everyone else ate honey and wax candles were also made from it. Mead, the traditional drink of the British, was based on honey, and there were very many different brews, most of which had health giving properties.'

'Tell me about it as an aphrodisiac,' Tana begged.

'Well, all the sacrificial wine used in the temples of different gods the world over had a base of honey. The most famous of the meads which was brewed in Ancient Greece by the great Galen was recorded as depressing anger, melancholia, sadness and all afflictions of the mind. Pleny wrote of it: 'It is well suited to persons of a chilly temperament.''

'I must try it on John,' Tana said with a smile.

'I told a meeting of women how to use it,' I said, 'and afterwards one wrote to me saying: 'Miss Cartland, I did what you suggested. I gave my husband honey and it works!' But, to return to the past, in *The Perfumed Garden*, a manual of Arabian erotology, by Sheik Nefzawi, who wrote it at the beginning of the sixteenth century, there is a poem translated by Sir Richard Burton. It extols the extraordinary vigour of an Arab hero who made love to 80 virgins in one night, and goes on:

> *"Now his diet before he united with these,*
> *Was honey and milk and ripe pigeon peas."*

'Perhaps it isn't such a good idea to give it to one's husband,' Tana laughed.

'In the East honey was indispensable,' I went on. 'All those sweetmeats on which the harem beauties gorged themselves were mixed with honey. And a special drink given to the bride and bridegroom on their wedding night was invariably a concoction of honey and herbs.'

'I suppose we haven't kept the recipe?' Tana asked wistfully.

'I'm afraid not, but I dare say I could make you one very nearly as good,' I replied. 'In the Greek and Roman civilisations honey was used for preserving and embalm-

27

ing as well as for the choicest dishes. What is so interesting – and do listen to this, Tana – is that in India
the healers used an ancient mixture known as Ceromel
for healing ulcers. It consisted of one part of beeswax
to four of honey. Only recently a doctor in Colorado
Agricultural College in the U.S.A., experimented with
putting various diseased bacteria into a pure honey
media. Within a few hours all the micro organisms were
dead. Typhoid fever producing germs died within forty-
eight hours; similar types known as A and B typhos
died within twenty-four hours.'

'I must say that is interesting,' Tana said. 'I was always
told that Cleopatra put honey on her face.'

'She did, and I'm going to tell you about honey for the
face a little later on,' I said. 'At the moment we are
trying to get your brain right. I believe that to get the
continual energy so that your brain is always active,
balanced and improving, – for your brain should improve as you get older, not, as so often happens,
deteriorate – you need honey.'

'How much?' Tana asked.

'Lots,' I answered. 'I have honey for breakfast, honey
for tea and honey last thing at night. But I also insist in
my household that fruit, cakes and ice cream are cooked
with honey; so altogether we have a great deal of honey
and we all feel amazingly well.'

'You all look it,' Tana said enviously.

'After the Olympic Games in Tokyo in 1964,' I continued, 'Miss Hartman, who was in charge of the British
women athletes, said to me: 'Miss Cartland, I thought
of you every day in Tokyo.'

'I'm flattered,' I replied, 'but why?'

'We always had honey on the breakfast table,' she answered.

'I laughed and said that was why we'd done so well that year. Mountain climbers, like Sir Edmund Hillary, swear by honey. In fact, when he reached the top of Mount Everest, his father, who was a bee-keeper in New Zealand, said: 'It's all been done on honey.''

'And you are sure it makes on live longer?' Tana asked.

'Longer and younger,' I replied. 'In 1623 Charles Butler, in 'The History of Bees' wrote: 'Honey clears all the obstructions of the body, loosens the belly, purges the foulness of the body and provoketh urine. It breedeth good blood and prolongeth old age.' In Ancient Greece it was thought that if the correct combination of food could be found the life span could be doubled. They regarded honey as a Youth Elixir, and the most important food of all. So you see, if you want to keep young and keep your brain agile you have got to take a lot of honey every day.'

'And I shall live to be a million!' Tana exclaimed.

'If you want to!' I replied. 'Pythagaros, who loved honey, invented a special drink made of milk and honey which was called 'ambrosia', of which, of course, you have read. He supplemented it with fruit, nuts and vegetables, the forerunner of our wonderful mueslis, and lived to be ninety. But a follower of his, called Appolonious, who also enjoyed this natural diet, lived to be one-hundred-and-five; while Piast, who was a bee-keeper and later became King of Poland in A.D. 824, lived until he was one-hundred-and-twenty-four.'

29

'With all this history about honey,' Tana remarked, 'it seems extraordinary to me that people don't realise the value of it. I suppose they have always been brought up to eat white sugar. It's easier, it's in a packet and it isn't so sticky.'

'Yet, arthritis, migraine, heart trouble and internal ulcers,' I went on, 'all get better, if you eat honey. I met a woman who had been in a wheel-chair for three years with rheumatism and she said to me: 'I ate half-a-pound of honey every day and now I can twist.' If, instead of taking those chemically produced drugs and anti-biotics, which often leave people far worse with side effects, they would try honey when they first get ill, stiff or in pain, they would get well so much quicker.'

'When I was young, I was told that the bees were part of the family and had to be told everything that happened,' Tana said.

'That's quite true,' I answered. 'When I was a little girl I believed, like all the country folk around my home, that if you didn't tell the bees what was happening in the household they would fly away and you would be terribly unlucky. If someone died, the country people in Worcestershire, used to go and knock on the beehive and say: 'So and so is dead!''

'It's fascinating,' Tana said. 'I suppose one of the reasons people don't value honey today is because it's cheap.'

'People only value things they can gauge in terms of money,' I said. 'If we were wise we would package honey in a special pot, call it an Elixir for the mind,

body and soul and sell it for £10. I believe we would
have an immense amount of customers.'

'You would have to prove it improved the mind,' Tana
said.

'What better proof than that of the Bible,' I replied.
'King Solomon, in the Book of Proverbs, says:— 'Son,
eat thou honey because it is good, and the honeycomb,
which is sweet to thy taste. So shall the knowledge of
wisdom be unto thy soul.''

'You have convined me,' Tana said. 'Honey from now
on and no sugar!'

'And you'll be as beautiful as the women in the Song
of Solomon,' I smiled. 'Because one of the experimental
places in Florida was run by a Dr. Page, and he noticed
that in both men and women, if they eliminated sugar
they not only lost weight, if they were over-weight to
start with, but the lines of their face took on a much
more handsome appearance. He said it was most un-
canny what the mere cutting out of sugar would do to
the face. So you see, Tana, not only will your brain be
active and intelligent but your face will be beautiful.
Could any woman ask more?'

'I've got a lot more to ask,' Tana said. 'Don't forget,
you've only got as far as my brain. There's all the rest.'

'Of course there is,' I said. 'But we have made a good
start.'

'And there is a great deal more I want to hear about
love,' Tana said eagerly.

CHAPTER III

The Body

'Where have we got to?' Tana asked the following afternoon, throwing herself down on the sofa looking extremely attractive in a pink wool dress with a gold belt. 'The next thing we must tackle,' I answered, 'is your body. We get so used to our bodies that we don't realise they are the most wonderful piece of mechanism that has ever been devised. If you really begin to think about a body, one is astounded that anyone could have thought of such a complex and yet, at the same time, such a simple machine!'

'Why simple?' Tana asked.

'Because it works! You don't have to think about it. You talk; you walk; you make gestures; you dance; you sing; you run upstairs. All the time there is an instinctive reflex from your mind sending orders to your limbs while you are apparently completely occupied with the ordinary details of a busy life.'

'I suppose it is really rather amazing,' Tana granted.

'When you think that your body is made up of thirty billion cells,' I told her, 'the thing which absolutely astounds me is that any of us are ever well or that we ever manage to get through life without being desperately ill almost the whole time. But, what is so stupid, is that we forget that these cells — the thirty billion of them — have to be supplied with oxygen and nutrition derived from the blood-stream, and they must be taken care of otherwise they weaken and die. Often, whole groups of cells deteriorate and cease to function and this means disease, unless these cells can be regenerated.'

'I don't like to think about it,' Tana said.

'Well, you've got to. And that is why we get back to the same old story that we have to feed every single cell of our body every day, otherwise this miraculous, fantastic machine will begin to break down and, eventually, die.'

Tana shuddered.

'And what is so frightening,' I went on, 'is that people don't appreciate a healthy body. Sometimes, when I visit hospitals where there are malformed and mentally retarded children, I go home thinking how deeply grateful we should be for not being born with some ghastly deformity. Think about the blind babies, the spastics, the mongols, the children crippled by polio, and realise that your body is something very precious and you must protect it.'

'How do I do that?' Tana asked.

'Well, the first thing, I believe, is good feeding, and the second is cleanliness. I often wonder how many diseases in the world have been started just because people are unclean. And you know, the British, as a race, are dirty.'

'I'm sure people would be furious with you for saying that,' Tana said.

'I'm sorry, but it's true,' I answered. 'You only have to go into our towns, big and small, and see the dirty, slum-like streets, which started as being quite respectable but have deteriorated merely because people don't take any interest. Nowadays, especially, when the ordinary person relies on some higher authority to do everything for them, they will hardly bother to put in a nail in a falling door or mend a broken gutter themselves. Visit a public lavatory or one on a crowded train; peep into the kitchens of small cafés or tea shops. You will be appalled! And, in the countryside, you have only got to look at the filthy litter which accumulates on every hedgerow, on every grass verge, in every little lane, to realise that English people have no respect for the beauty of the land.'

'I think that is very sweeping,' Tana said.

'Of course it's sweeping,' I said. 'One generalises! But, just go and look at a race-course after the race-goers have left, or a football ground after a match, and you'll be astounded at the tons and tons and tons of litter that has to be removed, usually at great expense. But, apart from all that, people are not clean in their houses. Go to almost any hotel that is not in the luxury class and see what the carpets are like, look at the dust that's accumulated in every room. You know, as well as I do, that wouldn't happen if people didn't put up with it. If people complained more about the dirt in rooms they rent or the chipped china off which they have to eat in restaurants, things would get cleaned up.'

'Your daughter made headlines because she complained about the dirt at London Airport,' Tana laughed.

'Quite rightly, too,' I said. 'I went to London Airport myself last year, on a Sunday, to fly to Glasgow to be on a television show, and I've never seen anything like the dirt on the only place there was to wait until the aeroplane came in. It isn't the fault of the London Airport authorities, it is the fault of travellers. They throw their cigarettes on the floor and stamp on them rather than put them in the ashtrays. They eat sweets and throw the wrappings away without making any attempt even to put them in the saucer on the table. They spill their tea; they drop food off their plates; and it really is the labour of Hercules to clean up after them. And yet, individually, I am sure they are all charming and delightful. It's just that they have never learned to be tidy and clean and one just wonders what their bodies are like.'

'You meant they don't wash?' Tana asked.

'I'm afraid that's still true of a great number of people,' I answered. 'Nowadays, a bathroom is essential in every house, but I often wonder how many people take a bath every day, let alone twice a day. In a recent survey of a wide diversity of people – M.P.s, television artistes, professional men, shop-keepers – it was found seven out of twenty bathed only once a week.'

'I think many people still believe that bathing is weakening,' Tana said.

'That really is an old wife's tale,' I laughed. 'I suppose if people had the time to lie in a hot bath for hours on end it might be enervating, but having a bath twice a day is not nearly as weakening as central heating.'

'I always have a bath once a day,' Tana said. 'But I prefer it in the morning.'

'I hate washing in a basin,' I replied. 'I love a bath even if it's just a quick splash in and out. But I do understand that men and women who have to rush to catch a train sometimes skimp their washing. But at night it is

35

essential to wash off the dirt that you have accumulated during the day, in the office, in the factory or even in ordinary rooms which are hot and which have made you sweat more than you realise.'

'I can't believe that anybody need suffer from B.O. these days,' Tana said, 'when every advertisement tells you how to avoid it.'

'I don't smoke,' I answered, 'so I'm afraid I notice that a lot of people, quite frankly, smell.'

'What do you advocate that they should do about it?' Tana asked.

'Well, washing is the first thing, and I think it is important for people who are fat, or athletic, or inclined to sweat in one way or another, that they should close their pores after a bath by a quick splashing of cold water over themselves or a rub-over with some type of astringent. There are hundreds of them on the market — eau de colognes of all sorts, or skin tonics, as they are now called — and all of them close up the pores and tighten up the skin. Incidentally, for women who want to keep their breasts a good shape there is nothing better than using an astrigent after a warm bath.'

'I shall remember that,' Tana said.

'There's an amusing story,' I went on, 'of two European Royalty, mother and daughter, escaping from Greece with the British Embassy as the Germans invaded it. They got as far as Crete the first night and stayed in a small, primitive hotel. No-one in the party thought of anything except how grateful they were to be safe, but in the morning the Royal mother of the beautiful young Princess was heard to say, plaintively, over and over again, 'I simply must have ice for my daughter's breasts'!!'

'Did she get it?' Tana asked.

'I'm sure she did,' I replied. 'But there's something I must tell you. I find that men and women who take vitamins, do not smell after a time. This makes me think that body odour comes from some deficiency. I noticed it particularly with a young man who had suffered with various skin complaints and smelt very unpleasantly after sleeping and exercise. After he had taken Bio-Strath, a herbal extract I will tell you about later, he ceased to smell.'

'Isn't there something called Chlorophyll?' Tana asked.

'Of course, there is,' I answered. 'Buy it in the form of *Amplex*. Two tablets take away all body smell, bad breath, etc. for two or three hours. Every girl who wants to be kissed should take Amplex before she goes out to dinner.'

'What next?' Tana enquired.

'If you're clean outside you obviously must be clean inside,' I replied. 'And we all know that the setting sin of the whole British nation is constipation. Ask any doctor and he'll tell you that numbers of his patients who have headache, skin troubles, feel limp and exhausted and are bad sleepers are invariably constipated, which is the root of the whole trouble. I taught my children when they were very young that one of the most important things in life is to get rid of the poisons that accumulate in the body. If you do not have a bowel movement every twelve hours, then the toxic poisonings that accumulate in the bowel begin to spread.'

'I'm sure that's right,' Tana murmured, 'but I often meet people who say that they go for days without going to the lavatory.'

'Those are the people who I'm quite certain end up with every sort of disease that it's possible to have,' I replied. 'And I never can understand why, if they are constipated to that extent, they don't do something about it.'

'I suppose they don't know what to do,' Tana said.

'Well, again we get back to right feeding,' I said. 'And it's not a question of just stuffing oneself with fruit, which can often have the opposite effect and upset people's digestion. I'm very wary of a lot of fruit because I find that people in this country are inclined to eat an enormous amount of plums, damsons or apples when they first come into season; then they are surprised that their digestion is upset and they get diarrhoea. I'm a great believer in herbs, and these, I think, are the right aperient for anyone who is constipated.'

'What sort of herbs?' Tana asked curiously.

'Well, personally, I take Culpeper's Aperient Tea last thing at night,' I said. 'To make it as simple as possible, I have a double spoon into which I put a small amount of the herbs. I pour boiling water on it when I go up to have my bath and change my clothes before the evening meal, then I drink it cold last thing at night when I go to bed. It has a very soft and soothing effect but it really does eliminate all the toxic poisons. I find that after taking Culpeper's Aperient Tea I have a bowel movement almost exactly eight hours later.'

'Surely that's rather a bother if one's in a hurry?' Tana

asked.

'One should never be in too much of a hurry to look after one's body,' I replied. 'But, when I'm travelling, I take with me a dry herbal mixture – there are plenty of them and, personally, I use Golden Lion herbs or Inner Fresh from Healthcrafts. I just put half a small spoonful in my mouth and wash it down with water; it's as easy as that. But I consider it is one of the most important things in my luggage and I would never, never travel without it.'

'I find aperients often give me terrible stomach pains,' Tana complained.

'Then try something quite new called Bio Vax. It's a suppository. Oh, I know English people hate suppositories but these give a normal evacuation and help re-educate your inside.'

'It's a clever idea,' Tana conceded, 'but just to get back to baths for a moment. Don't you find that hard water is very bad on the skin?'

'I was just going to talk about your skin,' I said. 'You see, people are always complaining to me that they have bad skin, not only on their face but on their body. It's rough and it has patches of irritation, or even, with some people, they itch all over. Now this, I am absolutely convinced, is entirely a vitamin deficiency. If you have very hard water it is quite easy, of course, to put a few drops of bath oil in it or, cheaper still, do what my children's Nanny always did, which was to use ordinary oatmeal sewn up into a bag and used, perhaps, a dozen times before it was thrown away. But, as a general rule, one's skin can stand up to the hard water and lots of other hardships without encountering the least damage if one is taking the right amount of vitamins.'

'That's funny,' Tana said, 'because I was thinking only the other day, after you had given me some vitamins, how much softer my skin was. In fact, my husband noticed it.'

'All women should have soft skin which is lovely to touch,' I answered. 'There was once a very famous beauty in London who had a very notorious career, and a man I knew very well was one of her great admirers. I said to him once:

'As we are old friends I am going to ask you a question. What was it that Doris did that attracted men so tremendously? Far more than the average woman.'

'He laughed and answered:

'"There were two things. First of all, she was at her very best and most charming when she was being made love to, because she enjoyed it so much. And, secondly, she had a skin which was so soft it was like touching the petals of a flower.' I think, perhaps, we would all like that said about us.'

'I suppose the fact is,' Tana said, 'that we don't think enough about our skins. You worry about your face but you never wonder if your hands are nice to touch.'

'It's traditional that a British woman always forgets her neck and hands,' I replied. 'Your neck is one of the first tell-tale signs of age and all that crepiness can be prevented if you use a good nourishing cream on your neck every night.'

Tana looked guilty.

'I always feel it's rather extravagant to use my best face

cream on my neck,' she confessed.

I threw back my head and laughed.

'Everybody has a meanness,' I said, 'and I'm sure that's quite a common one. But it really is a false economy. If your face looks lovely and it's supported by an ugly, old, wrinkled neck you are not going to look very young.'

'No, you are quite right,' Tana said. 'In future I shall be more extravagant.'

'I think it may be wrong to use the same cream on your face as on your neck,' I said. 'Because I believe your neck needs a far heavier cream and I don't really approve of very heavy nourishing creams on the face – not very often. They are making them much lighter nowadays and one of the best I've found is Celaton's Night Star. This refines my skin and my face is smooth and flawless in the morning. Another I like enormously is Zodiac's Face Conditioning Cream. This tightens the skin naturally and also gives a flawless appearance the next morning. After this cream and any other, I always use Celaton's Moisturising Cream as soon as I wake up.'

'I must make a note of those,' Tana cried.

'No, don't bother,' I replied. 'I'm not going to talk about your face for the moment. I want to concentrate on your body as a whole. Now, we've talked about having baths, and not being constipated but we haven't yet mentioned that posture is one of the most important things in being young and beautiful. Just watch the average middle-aged woman walking down the street.'

'I have,' Tana said, 'and it's horrifying!'

'You see how they begin to walk with their behinds sticking out and their necks stuck forward,' I said. 'Now, one of the easiest ways to get your right posture is to walk about on tip-toe. I always recommend it for busy people who never seem to have time for exercises.'

'On tip-toe?' Tana queried.

'Just try it,' I said. 'Stand up on your toes and you'll see how it pulls in your tummy, lifts your head and takes away that arch in your back which is so unbecoming.'

Tana kicked off her shoes, raised herself on her toes, and looked at herself in one of the long mirrors which hang on my drawing-room wall.

'You're right!' she exclaimed. 'It makes me look much slimmer.'

'Of course it does,' I said, 'because you're lifting your chest and lengthening your waist. One of the most boring things about getting old is that you begin to lose your waist. Now that you are pulling yourself up you see the difference. From having a rather stolid, old body, you have a young, streamlined one.'

'But, I can't permanently walk about like this,' Tana said, admiring herself from every angle.

'You can,' I replied. 'You've got to go on walking like that even when you're not on tip-toe.'

'I can't keep thinking about it,' Tana said.

'Of course, you can't,' I agreed. 'We are all too busy. But, whenever you can, walk on tip-toe and feel your body lengthening itself into a young look. When you walk across your bedroom, walk on tip-toe; as you undress, do it on tip-toe; as you do your housework, you can do that on tip-toe too.'

Tana groaned.

'I shan't remember,' she said.

'You must try,' I said firmly. 'Do you know, I had a friend who, when she was over sixty-five, determined to slim her waist. So, every day she raised her hands above her head and tried to see how high she could stretch. She would stretch up with her right hand and then the left, and make it go higher, and so on. She took two inches off her waist in a month. It does work! Granted, she had time to do it; but you can try, once a day, if possible, and at the week-end, to improve your figure. There's nothing really more depressing than that middle-age spread.'

'I'm so terrified of having it,' Tana said. 'It's the one thing that makes me start slimming.'

I gave a little groan.

'Why do you do that?' Tana enquired.

'Because we've got to the most depressing subject of all,' I said. 'Slimming! Now, it's something on which I have very, very strong views.'

'Which are – not to do it, I suppose,' Tana said tartly.

'No! To do it the right way,' I corrected. 'I'll confess that I am very against women slimming in a haphazard manner. I've see such tragedies. There was a friend of mine – actually I was at school with her – who I hadn't seen for years. I asked after her last week. I found that about ten years ago she started slimming. She has made herself so ill that she is now nothing more nor less than a chronic invalid. I know another young girl who was determined to get slim and she went to fantastic lengths to eat so little that in the end she couldn't eat at all and she, too, nearly died. She has just got married and her secret fear is that because she did this crazy, unintelligent slimming and made herself so ill, she will never be able to have a baby. People are insane the way they torture their bodies, simply because they think it will make them more beautiful.'

'But, you know yourself, none of us want to be fat,' Tana answered.

'Of course, you don't,' I said. 'At the same time, you're not going to be beautiful or attractive if you're neurotic, nervy, disagreeable and irritable. And that's what happens to most women when they slim. They also, generally, look awful. It's no use having a slim figure and a lined, ugly face.'

'No, of course not,' Tana said, rather doubtfully.

'What you have got to decide, first of all, is who you are slimming for and for what reason,' I said. 'You see, I've never yet met a man who didn't like an armful!'

Tana laughed.

'That's true,' she said. 'John is always saying to me: ''You're very nice as you are; I like plump women.''

'I've yet to find the man who liked a thin one,' I said. 'So woman are really doing it to please other women and, perhaps, pansy dressmakers who want one to look like a boy! Now, the first thing you have got to do, before you slim, is to look at yourself in the glass. Most women will find that they have round, unlined faces looking much younger than their years but beneath it, of course, their body is plump in the wrong places. Their hips have got broad; they have a tummy; and a large number will have what is known as a 'spare tyre'.'

'You can't say that's pretty,' Tana said.

'No, of course, it isn't,' I answered. 'But, at the same time, I find with so many women of this sort that they are full of vitality, full of charm, that they have energy to do a dozen jobs and that their husbands and children adore them.'

'Because they are fat?' Tana said doubtfully.

'Because they have that little extra protection which keeps them good tempered and full of vitality,' I answered. 'Now, it's not worth losing all that on the credit side to be thin. But, they can lose a certain amount of inches without harming themselves.'

'But, how?' Tana asked.

'Well, of course, you'll moan when I tell you that it's diet,' I said. 'It's no use my letting you believe that there is a magic pill which will enable you to eat everything you want to eat and not put on weight. It has just not been invented. I've tried all sorts of slimming diets – because I never recommend anything that I haven't tried myself – and the majority follow exactly the same pattern. I take the pills, or drink the liquids – whichever it may be; I cut out all the things which make meals interesting and amusing; and I drop weight. But, within three weeks I have a bout of 'flu and, because I feel so ill, I eat – and on goes all the weight again!'

'You are depressing,' Tana said.

'In any womens' magazine you pick up you will find slimming diets. Most af them are extremely bad for you because they recommend a lot of citrus fruit, which your digestion usually cannot stand, and black coffee, which we know is very bad and which makes your hair

45

go grey.'

'Why,' Tana asked.

'Because coffee destroys Vitamin B,' I replied. 'In an experiment in the U.S.A. they added coffee to the food of sleek, young, well-fed rats. Within a week they began to show every sign of Vitamin B deficiency. They went grey; their hair and teeth fell out; they were quarrelsome and they went sterile.'

'Go on, tell me your diet,' Tana said.

'There is only one diet on which you will feel wonderful and on which you will lose weight,'* I said. 'It is, I regret to say, deadly dull, but that is the self-discipline you must impose on yourself if you care enough about your figure.'

'Well, tell it to me,' Tana said.

'This is it,' I replied.

Breakfast: 1 or 2 boiled eggs; 2 teaspoonsful of honey; weak tea without milk or sugar.

Lunch: Half-pound of steak or a large helping of meat and green vegetables; one small piece of unprocessed cheese.

Tea: 1 cup of weak tea, no milk or sugar; 2 teaspoonsful of honey.

Dinner: A small piece of fish or a cup of clear soup; half-pound of steak and green vegetables, or the equivalent amount of other meat.

6 teaspoons of sunflower oil spread over the day.

* Margin Note: Since writing this I have heard of a 'Magic Slimming Diet' based on research by the Mayo Clinic. I have tried it and it is included at the back of the book.

'Now, nothing, nothing, nothing else is permitted! But you must eat everything I have listed. You can drink water at lunch and water at supper, or, if you prefer, you can have tea at both those meals; no coffee, no alcohol. You will lose weight but it is very boring and, of course, I don't need to say, that at the same time, you must take your vitamins – and quite a lot of them!'

'They're not fattening, are they?' Tana asked.

'I suppose I'm asked that question at least a thousand times a month,' I replied. 'No! No! No! Natural Vitamins are food but they're not fattening. The only way they affect your appetite is that they balance your body so that you're naturally healthy and naturally hungry at the right time. But, they do not over-stimulate the appetite and no vitamin is fattening in itself, any more than honey is fattening. Sugar is desparately fattening in every form; but, honey – which is pre-digested by the bee – is not fattening except in very abnormal quantities. And, when people ask me if honey is fattening, it usually means that they eat it with bread and butter, in which case it is the bread which is fattening and not the honey.'

Tana looked depressed.

'I know it's a deadly diet,' I said, 'and if you're sensible you will not, at your age, try and get too thin. To begin with, you are not going to look like Twiggy – whatever you do to yourself! And, secondly, it's very unbecoming if you begin to get those lines on either side of your mouthand a scraggy neck, because, however much you may try, if you slim it always affects the face. With older people who are not so elastic as the

47

young, the skin doesn't tighten up so quickly, if at all. So, if you are not careful, you will get a sagging chin.'

Tana looked unconvinced and I went on:

'I saw a horrible sight the other day. A woman who had really been very beautiful in her youth had decided that she would slim. I saw her back view first of all and I thought what a good figure she had; and then, when she turned round, I saw that her face, which had once been so lovely, was wrinkled all over like Chinese parchment. She really looked quite hideous and I couldn't imagine why she thought it was worth the sacrifice of her face to keep her figure.'

'Well, that's silly, of course,' Tana said. 'At the same time, you said, yourself, that nothing is worse than a middle-age spread.'

'A lot of that comes from walking badly and sitting badly,' I said. 'A few months ago Zena Dare came down to lunch with me in the country. She's over eighty and has the figure of a young girl. As I watched her I realised why she looked so young and had kept her figure so wonderfully. It was not through dieting but through posture. She walked so erect and yet so gracefully and when she sat down she never slouched in her chair. She sat upright with her back straight and you know that that is important. They always say that Queen Mary had the most wonderful digestion because she held herself so regally – always with a straight back.'

'It's awfully difficult to sit without slouching, in modern chairs and sofas,' Tana said.

'I agree with you there,' I replied. 'I've got long legs and when I'm on the television I am always having trouble with those low, modern chairs they have on the sets. I usually have to demand a telephone book – or even a sandbag on one or two occasions! – on which I can perch myself so that I don't thrust forward my tummy and curl up, like a pocket knife. And I'm quite convinced that a large number of women lose their figures simply because they sit badly, more than for any other reason.'

'I quite see that I shall have to buy a new set of furniture,' Tana said.

'No, just sit on the edge of your chair,' I suggested. 'And in the dining-room where the chairs are upright, do try and sit with your tummy held in and your shoulders back. You'll be surprised what a difference it makes to your digestion. And, also, there's one other tip I'd like to give you and one which my Mother firmly believes is essential to a good digestion.'

'What is that?' Tana asked.

'Drink at the end of a meal,' I answered. 'We all know that it's slimming to drink between meals but I always think that's an awful bother and one forgets. But my Mother was brought up never to drink during a meal; she drinks at the end – with the result that at ninety she has the most elegant figure and can wear a riding habit which she wore when she was eighteen.'

'I wonder if that really does affect the figure,' Tana asked.

'I think it does,' I replied. 'And I'll tell you something else. I find that if one eats a dry meal one eats less. It's very easy to wash down food with a drink. And, while we're talking of drinking, I regret to tell you that the one thing which really stimulates the appetite and which you must give up if you want to slim, is a drink before a meal. A glass of sherry, a cocktail, or even a non-alcoholic drink, does stimulate the digestive juices and make you hungrier when you go into the dining-room. So, if you want to keep slim, that's out!'

'It's a most depressing thought that everything that's nice is forbidden,' Tana said.

'It's illegal, it's immoral or it makes you fat,' I quoted. 'That's why I say, enjoy yourself and don't worry too much about being thin. You can slim sensibly. If you're alone at home you can eat a piece of cold meat and nothing else. You won't feel tired and you certainly won't put on weight. When you're out, eat what is put in front of you. There's nothing more infuriating to a hostess than to plan a wonderful meal and then have somebody say they're dieting and peck away at a lettuce leaf!'

'I suppose we all eat too much,' Tana said.

'On the contrary, most people eat too little and what they do eat is wrong,' I answered. 'Most people's bodies are suffering from mal-nutrition. It hardly seems possible, in this day and age, when the majority of people have more money than they have ever had before; but, it's true. They did a research in Pennsylvania, in America, six years ago, and they found that only one person in a thousand was not vitamin deficient. And in this country they have found that millions of people are definitely under-nourished although they are eating three meals a day.'

'It seems incredible,' Tana said.

'It does! At the same time, you don't want to add to their number,' I said. 'There always seems to me something rather horrible about women who have money, deliberately becoming under-nourished when there are millions of people in India on the verge of starvation simply because they cannot get food of any sort!'

'But, does it hurt you to give up a meal occasionally?'

'I think it's a stupid thing to do,' I said. 'And that is where people who are slimming are so idiotic. They imagine that by eating nothing they will get slim. They don't! It merely makes them feel ill, because their blood sugar, about which I've already explained, drops very low. This gives them headaches and a feeling of exhaustion, which is definitely very ageing.'

'If you are going to diet you must do it properly, eating exactly what I've told you at every meal and, preferably, at exactly the same time every day. You are using your body and it's got to have the nourishment on which to work. To deprive it for long hours on end of food of any sort is, definitely, to damage yourself. Also it uses up nervous energy, which we know to have very bad repercussions mentally.'

'There seem to be so many snags,' Tana said.

'There aren't really,' I replied. 'Think of your body as a machine. Don't think of it as something which can be ill treated by you because it belongs to you. It's a machine which you've got to keep going at a proper speed and for that it requires the nutriment which you would give to any normal machine. You wouldn't expect your car to go without oil, petrol and water. Therefore, your body required food and liquid in exactly the same way – otherwise it just won't go! You know as well as I do that if you have a very expensive car and one small part of it breaks down, then the whole thing comes to a stand-still. Well, it's just the same as your body; refuse to feed one small part and the whole of your body will be affected.'

Tana looked pensive.

'You know, you are right,' she said. 'The body is a very, very wonderful invention!'

CHAPTER IV

'The Milk of Human Kindness'

'I've done such a silly thing,' Tana said when she arrived at my house. 'I put a book I wanted to give you on the hall table and then I forgot it.'

'Bring it tomorrow,' I said.

'I hope I don't forget,' Tana replied. 'I've been so forgetful lately. You won't believe it, but I got into a taxi yesterday in a hurry and then couldn't remember where I was going. The taxi-driver said: 'Well, where's it to be? twice round the Serpentine or a trip to the moon?' I did feel a fool and it was two or three minutes before I remembered that I had an appointment at the dentist.'

'Lack of Vitamin B,' I smiled.

'Is it, really?' Tana asked. 'Is it dangerous to be short of vitamin B?'

'It is very ageing and it can be expensive,' I replied. 'A friend of mine was going away for the week-end and at the last moment she found she had left out her diamond ring. She wrapped it in a face tissue and put it in her handbag. In the train, seeing a crumpled tissue, she threw it out of the window!'

'I hope I won't do anything as silly as that,' Tana said.

'It's exactly the same as forgetting your address,' I told her. 'So let us start on the various vitamins which affect your health. The most important vitamin of all is vitamin B. I suppose you know it is called 'the milk of human kindness'?'

'I didn't,' Tana said. 'Why?'

'Well, a lack of thiamine, which is the correct word for vitamin B_1, results in personality changes which are frightening,' I answered. 'A gay, happy person can suddenly become irritable and depressed. They can also develop nerves, skin diseases, muscular weakness and hives.'

'It sounds like Jekyll and Hyde,' Tana said.

'It is worse,' I answered, 'because so many people do not realise what is happening to themselves. A woman will quarrel with her husband, sometimes fatally so that it leads to the Divorce Courts. She will lose the affection and trust of her children and find herself growing old, without friends.'

'Good heavens!' Tana exclaimed. 'You'd better tell me how much I must take.'

'I will,' I replied, 'but first of all, I want you to understand about vitamin B. Do you remember how ill the Allied prisoners were who were in the hands of the Japanese? Many of the men who worked on the Burma Road died from beri-beri, which is a terrible disease caused by lack of vitamins, especially vitamin B.'

'Which is the best way to take it?' Tana asked.

'Well, the cheapest way,' I answered, 'is in Brewers' Yeast, which contains all the elements of vitamin B complex. It's so cheap that the cost of 250 tablets is only 3/9d., and when I talk to old age pensioners, I always suggest to them that they eat honey – instead of that mucky marmalade, which has never seen an orange, or cheap jam, which has never seen any fruit – and that they buy themselves Brewers' Yeast tablets instead of cigarettes. It's absolutely amazing the difference that these two things can make to them.'

'Why is Brewers' Yeast so good?' Tana asked.

'Well, yeast is the smallest of all cultivated plants – about 1–4,000th of an inch in diameter – but it has the strength of a giant when it is absorbed in the body. Since the days of the early Egyptians mankind has used yeast for making and brewing.'

'I suppose I can get Brewers' Yeast from a brewery?' Tana asked.

'You can, but I don't advise people taking the Brewers' Yeast which is obtained from the brewery,' I answered, 'although I used to give it to my pigs!'

'Your pigs!' Tana exclaimed.

'Yes, I realised how important vitamins were, not only to us but to animals,' I said. 'And when I had 52 far-rowing sows I had the most amazing litters – an average of twelve per sow for two or three years – and it was entirely because I used to fetch, twice a week, an enormous tin bath full of Brewers' Yeast from our local brewery. In face, I was so successful that Sir Harry Haig, who kept a large number of pigs on his Ovaltine farms, copied my way of looking after the sows, and, of course, the boars, who had Brewers' Yeast as well.'

'Why did your pigs want it?' Tana asked.

'Well, it not only produced enormous litters,' I said, 'but it also gave the sows plenty of milk. It is the best and easiest way to eat protein. Meat, fish and eggs are all essential to our health and to keep us young but we would have to eat very large quantities of these to equal the amount of protein in Brewers' Yeast.'

'And protein is essential to the cells of the body,' Tana said.

'You're learning quickly,' I laughed. 'Brewers' Yeast contains sixteen of the twenty amino acids and these are forms of protein which are essential for a long life, resistance to disease and the proper functioning of our bodies. One of the most important of the B complex vitamins B_2. A deficiency of this vitamin means sore and tired eyes, sores round the mouth and acute sensitivity to light.'

'My eyes do hurt me sometimes,' Tana said, 'I get a kind of gritty feeling in them.'

'That is lack of vitamin B_2,' I answered. 'You can take it singly, in capsule form – I always do as I am very fussy about eyes and I've see the marvellous results of vitamin B_2 on people with bad sight. But, for the average person, Brewers' Yeast every day is enough in itself, because you get the vitamin B_2 in it. A deficiency of Niacin, another of the B group, produces painful sores in the mouth and on the tongue, and also diarrhoea.'

'I'm beginning to think I have sores in the mouth when you talk about it,' Tana said.

'Take Brewers' Yeast,' I smiled. 'And let me tell you the strength of Brewers' Yeast compared to other high protein foods:–

FOOD	PARTS OF VITAMIN B_1 per 100 grams.
Brewers' Yeast	5,000 to 8,000
Kidney	1,700 to 2,200
Liver	1,800 to 2,200

'That seems pretty conclusive,' Tana said.

'Brewers' Yeast is, of course, highly concentrated,' I went on, 'in fact, three tablespoons of Brewers' Yeast weighs as much as an ordinary portion of liver.'

'If there's one thing I dislike, it's liver!' Tana exclaimed.

'But, it's very good for you,' I replied. 'And so are kidneys. I didn't used to like them, but if they are well cooked they are delicious. Try the Robert Carrier recipe of 'Kidneys Flambe'.'

'Is that with brandy?' Tana asked.

'It is,' I replied. 'But to return to Brewers' Yeast, two of the youngest and gayest of my friends are two very famous stage stars. She is the entrancing actress, Pat Kirkwood, and her husband is Hubert Gregg, who often acts with her. He has just written the most exciting and dramatic musical of Nell Gwyn – about which we are all going to hear a lot in the future as it will be a film and, I hope, performed on the stage at Drury Lane.'

'Pat and Hubert lunched with me the other day and when the meal ended they both took out little boxes, opened them and produced three small tablets. 'What are those?' I asked curiously. 'Brewers' Yeast tablets,' Pat replied. 'We always take them after every meal and we know they give us energy for the most exhausting rehearsals and performances. What is more, we seldom have colds!'

'She looked so pretty and glamorous as she spoke that I thought no-one could be a better advertisement for any product.'

'I admire Pat Kirkwood enormously,' Tana said. 'I shall certainly take Brewers' Yeast if she takes it.'

'Aren't women extraordinary?' I smiled. 'They always think the other woman has the elixir of youth! But actually, Pat is very wise. She also takes Bio-Strath, about which I'll tell you later. I just want to finish about vitamin B.'

'People are always complaining to me that they have no energy. 'I'm tired when I get out of bed!' they moan. This is a direct result of their food being robbed of the essential B vitamins, especially B_1 (thiamine).'

'I feel exhausted about six o'clock in the evening,' Tana said, 'just when John comes home. So I'm irritable and disagreeable when I plan to be so nice to him!'

'Take vitamin B before he arrives,' I suggested. 'There's a delicious new wheat germ called Kretschmers Wheatgerm with Raw Sugar and Honey. Wheatgerm is one of the best sources of vitamin E, iron and all the B vitamins. Take a few spoonsful at 5.30. You will greet John with open arms.'

'I shall do that,' Tana said. 'I think he will be surprised. What else contains vitamin B?'

'Black treacle,' I answered, and laughed at Tana's face. 'I can't bear it,' she protested.

'I agree with you,' I said. 'So stick to the wheat germ, or you can, if you want a change, mix powdered Brewers' Yeast with blackcurrant juice. I think it's better to make sure one has enough of this all important vitamin by taking it in tablet form. I find Liver Plus an excellent source and it makes one bound with energy! I gave it to some 'ton-up' boys and they told me they won all their races.'

I paused and said slowly:

'Vitamin B is absolutely essential to car drivers. I am sure that thousands of accidents could be prevented if drivers took it. Actually, I should have told you this when we were discussing the brain, for thiamine (B_1) is the activation of the food necessary to keep the brain healthy and alert, enabling it to make use of the oxygen in the bloodstream.'

'So, I'm forgetful because I need thiamine,' Tana summarised.

'Exactly,' I said. 'But it's really no use discussing deficiencies of the B group separately. They all go together and that is why I advise you to take Brewers' Yeast. Besides, remember that I told you it is a proven prevention against cancer.'

'I've heard people say that natural vitamins were a protection against cancer,' Tana said, 'but I was never quite sure I really believed it.'

'Well, I think we shall find that all sorts of vitamins not only prevent cancer but cure it,' I answered. 'But at the moment they have been proved to be a protection. Scientists are working, now, on vitamin A as a prevention to cancer and, here again, is a vitamin which I must tell you about because it is so essential to your looks and general health.'

'But, before we leave vitamin B, I want you to realise how important it is that one should not be short of this all-important vitamin. Lassitude, sleepiness, muscular pain, loss of appetite, pallor, dryness of the skin, a feeling of distress in the region of the heart and disturbances of the nervous system are all pointers to the fact that one is vitamin B deficient.'

'I expect I've got the lot,' Tana murmured.

'In animals,' I went on, ignoring the interruption, 'a peculiar loss of hair, called spectacle eye, results from a Biotin deficiency. The animals lose the hair round their eyes so that the bald rings of skin resemble spectacles. Baldness and sparcity also result in animals who do not obtain enough Biotin in their diet. And Biotin is very necessary for growing tissues so pregnant women and nursing mothers should also have plenty of Biotin in their diets. It is present in human breast milk. Scientists believe that Biotin may involve in the assimilation of fat or the carbohydrate in our bodies, and, here again, you get back to what is important if you want to keep slim.'

'In what sort of ordinary food do we get vitamin B?' Tana asked.

'Meat, liver, milk, eggs, molasses, mushrooms, salmon, chicken; in fact, practically everything that is good food has vitamin B in it,' I answered. 'And, before we leave vitamin B, I must mention Riboflavin again. I have, as I've already told you, found it wonderful for people with bad eyesight and it helps people with psoriasis, that terrible skin disease. Also, anyone who wants to have sparkling, gay eyes – like yours ought to be, Tana – must have Riboflavin (Vitamine B_2). Personally, I always take two vitamin B_2 capsules every day of my life and, since I have been doing it, although I wear glasses for reading, I have not had to have their strength increased for over six years.'

CHAPTER V

'The Life Vitamin'

'What's the next vitamin?' Tana asked, throwing herself down on my sofa. 'I feel exactly like a school girl again, coming here every day for my lessons. But I attend a good deal more than I did at school.'

'Well, I'm going to jump from B to E,' I said, 'because vitamin E, to my mind, is one of the most exciting and important vitamins that has yet been discovered.'

'I thought it was something to do with the menopause,' Tana said.

'It was, originally,' I replied, 'because during the war in the Japanese concentration camps in the Philippines, the only vitamin that the doctors had with them, for some unknown reason, was vitamin E. They gave this to the women who were suffering from the change of life and other female disorders and it had such an amazing effect on their general health that the doctors then tried it on men. They discovered that vitamin E is really the life vitamin. It is also the sex vitamin, and if you haven't got sex, you also haven't got much life, because you are old and, really, finished. And so vitamin E, to my mind, is the vitamin of life. I have seen the most amazing things in the last few years done with vitamin E.'

'Tell me about them,' Tana said.

'Well, it's achieved its greatest reputation in treating circulatory diseases and, because it could maintain a high level of oxygen in the blood, it is a tremendous help to people with heart diseases. But, it also turned out, that by taking oxygen into every part of the body and into every tissue, it also maintained the body's reproductive powers and slowing or halting completely the dissemination of certain organs of the body in old age. In other words, it keeps you young!'

'Tell me everything about it,' Tana begged.

'That is difficult,' I smiled, 'because what is so exciting about vitamin E is that they are always finding something new it cures.'

'Tell me what they have discovered already,' Tana insisted.

'Well, apart from heart patients who it has been proved to have helped over and over again,' I said, 'it also cures varicose veins. A friend of mine had had two operations on her legs for varicose veins and she said to me, 'I'm afraid I've got to have a third.' I said, 'Will you try vitamin E?' She replied: 'I'll try anything rather than have the operation again; I'm too busy, for one thing.' So, I made her take eight units of one hundred each, – in other words 800 units – of vitamin E every day. Not only did she not have to have the operation but her legs were so much better that you can hardly see the varicose veins through her stockings. What is more, she said it was so amazing the difference in her circulation.

'When I used to swim,' she told me, 'I always went blue. Now, I can swim for hours and my fingers are just the same as they are ordinarily.''

'I get goose pimples all over me when I bathe,' Tana interposed, but I continued,

'One of the French medical journals reported that 44 patients with types of varicose vein complaints were treated with 300 to 500 milligrams of vitamin E daily for two months to nine years. Nine of the cases of varicose ulcers showed improvement within thirty days – seven were complete cures – and the other 35 all showed some improvement.'

'Now, I spoke to Dr. Shute, myself, in Canada some years ago and he said the only thing about vitamin E was that you must take it in maximum doses. He said it was quite useless to take it in small amounts and that is why I and my sons take 1,000 milligrams every day.'

'Go on,' Tana encouraged, 'I'm absolutely rivetted!'

'A friend of mine,' I continued, 'came to me in deep distress because her boy, who was then fourteen, was so short. He was getting a terrible complex about it and he also hadn't reached puberty. I told her to give the boy 4 vitamin E capsules or, in other words, 400 milligrams, every day and within a very few weeks the boy had begun to grow; he soon reached puberty and was so much better and happier in himself that he was a delight to his parents.'

'Vitamin E, of course, is one of the things which prevents abortion and I think, myself, that it is always wise, when one is having a baby, to take vitamin E and Wheat Germ Oil together. Wheat Germ Oil was the first vitamin experimented with in the Distressed Areas after World War I and in 1948, after the last war, the conception rate of mares given vitamin E and serviced by prudent stallions was increased by 5 per cent and the number of live foals was increased by 7 per cent.

63

The number of still births, abortions and early losses in foals was reduced by 40 per cent when vitamin E was used. It was further remarked that the sex urge of the stallions was found to increase with the inclusion of vitamin E in their diet.'

'That should be interesting to all husbands,' Tana said.

'It should be interesting to all wives, too,' I replied, 'because women who feel frigid or disinterested in sex definitely feel very different when they, too, have taken vitamin E. And men who are impotent should take vitamin E in large doses.'

'Do most men know this?' Tana asked.

'Of course they don't,' I replied. 'Impotency is one of the things that is most hush-hush, because men cannot bear to think they are a failure. But, I will tell you more about that later on. At the moment, I want you to realise that vitamin E is something that every woman should take if she wants to remain young and beautiful.'

'I shall start tomorrow,' Tana cried.

'I think that vitamin E affects the skin tremendously,' I said. 'We know that it brings oxygen requirements to the tissues; it melts clots and in the case of acute phlebitis a clot may disappear in as little as five days; it increases collateral circulation; it helps the smaller blood vessels open up and so return the blood supply along alternative channels to the affected limbs or area; it dilates the capillaries which brings the blood and oxygen to the region where it is most needed; it occasionally removes excessive scar tissue and it prevents the over-production of it; it decreases the insulant requirement in diabetics and is one of the regulators of fat and protein metabolism!'

I paused for breath.

'Now, all these, in themselves,' I continued, 'add up to a healthy body. Therefore, I do feel that vitamin E is something which you must use if you want to keep well. There's only one time that you shouldn't take it and that is if you are taking artificial iron under the direction of a doctor. Actually, most doctors don't give iron these days; they give you B.12, which is the best possible way to prevent anaemia in any form. But if you do take vitamin E and ordinary iron, for some unknown reason the iron cancels out the vitamin E.'

'I'm most interested in why it stops you getting old,' Tana said.

'Well, all these things add up to youth,' I replied. 'But, Dr. Aloys Tappel, a biochemist at the University of California, has said that, in his opinion, vitamin E can definitely slow down the ageing process in humans. 'Ageing,' says Dr. Tappel, 'is due to the process of oxidation and since vitamin E is a natural anti-oxident, it can be used to counteract this process in the body.''

'I don't quite understand that,' Tana said.

'Well, when oxidation occurs in the body, the results are the formation of very high reaction compounds which may cause a breakdown and loss of the function of proteins which, as you know, build up the body. The debris from these destroyed proteins tends to pile up in cell membranes and accounts for the appearance and behaviour which are characteristic of ageing.'

'Dr. Tappel suggested that the extra vitamin E might be used in infancy to extend man's life span by decades.

An experiment based on Dr. Tappel's ideas was done in 1961 and they were able to extend the life of experimental mice by 20 per cent.'

'Now, no-one wants to live old just for the sake of being old, just as we've already said, Tana. But, I do believe that you will feel young and look younger if you take vitamin E. And, of course, you must have it to prevent any of those tiresome evidences of the menopause.'

'I do get hot flushes sometimes,' Tana said. 'Especially when I'm nervous or in a frantic hurry. I also feel ghastly at the time the period is due.'

'All this is quite unnecessary these days,' I said, 'I have found that when women have hot flushes, nerves, headaches, etc. if they will take 6–10 vitamin E each day, plus Bio-Strath No. 10, Feminal, they will find themselves being perfectly normal in every way and having no undue symptoms of their time of life.'

'I wish I had known this five years ago,' Tana said.

'Start at once,' I told her, 'and one tip that is very helpful is never eat fruit either just before or during the period.'

'Why?' Tana enquired.

'It's too acid,' I replied. 'And I can't tell you what a difference having no fruit makes to girls who have pains with their periods. They will never believe me until they have tried it.'

'Tell me more about vitamin E,' Tana begged.

'I believe that vitamin E is a prevention against many diseases,' I answered, 'as well as a cure.'

'Why should vitamin E have such remarkable powers? Even greater, it appears, than other vitamins,' Tana

asked.

'There has been one explanation given for this,' I replied. 'For many thousands of years human beings have eaten grains – it was, of course, after animals, the first food of man – and whole grains are the richest source of vitamin E, aside from vegetable oils. So, right down the ages many of today's most troublesome diseases were unknown; muscular dropsy, heart and blood vessel diseases, and so on. I don't say these are only caused by a deficiency of vitamin E – there are, undoubtedly, other reasons – but vitamin E does perform such miracles that I know that it is a vitamin I should hate to be without.'

'I must add to this, however, that it is important to take the other vitamins as well. Vitamin E therapy is enhanced by the addition of multi-vitamins and other substances. An American researcher in vitamin E likes people to also take B-complex, vitamin C with Bioflavods, dried liver tablets – in other words Brewers' Yeast – calcium and Wheat Germ Oil concentrate. He believes that vitamins work best in conjunction with each other and should never be taken alone because they may upset the metabolic balance or the dynamic equilibrium of a body.'

'It's a lot,' Tana complained.

'You also have a lot of body,' I replied sharply. 'But think of all these things as food. If you put all you eat during the day into a bucket, you would be astonished at how much you get through. All I'm asking you to swallow is a small handful of extra food.'

'I apologise,' Tana laughed.

'One other thing that I must tell you about vitamin E,' I said, 'is that it is a marvellous healer for burns and injuries. When used as an ingredient in ointment on a burn or a wound, and also taken internally, it has been found by no less than seven researchers in various countries to hasten the healing of the wound; and, most significantly, to reduce the amount of scar tissue in some cases.'

'In that case, surely, it would be wonderful as a face cream?' Tana said.

'Various firms are experimenting with this, I believe, but so far the only one I have tried is by Maria Hornes. Her cream contains vitamin E and B.12. But I can't repeat too often that vitamin E taken internally does clear the skin and give it a kind of glow which, of course, is obviously the oxygen surging all over the body.'

'What else does it help?' Tana asked.

'Arthritis, for one thing. I always recommend that people with arthritis and rheumatism should take vitamin E, as well as Bio-Strath Rheum-Elixir, B.12, vitamin A, Brewers' Yeast, vitamin B.6, lots of vitamin C and Bone Meal. Vitamin E improves the mobility of the joints; pain is reduced and, in some cases, absolutely eliminated.'

'Another discovery by Dr. Shute is that vitamin E, in sufficient doses, clears up and controls many forms of kidney disease. I used to have a little bit of trouble with my kidneys and since I have taken vitamin E, I seem to be cured. For one thing, vitamin E reduces excessive water in the kidneys and it also has a beneficial effect on the kidney cells themselves.'

'I shall remember that,' Tana said.

'One of the things which affects a great number of older women is that vitamin E helps swollen ankles, aching legs and knees. Women who work in shops often write to me and I always recommend that they take vitamin E and lecithin. I find that the two together really do help their legs and nothing is more depressing, when you lie down at night, than to feel them aching and throbbing so that you can't go to sleep.'

'I thought the doctors weren't very keen on vitamin E,' Tana said.

'Some doctors are still saying it's not proven, despite the millions of people all over the world who have found it of tremendous benefit,' I said. 'But, I can only tell you what I find for myself, and I have found that vitamin E not only makes me feel young, it helps my legs and it eliminates any sign of varicose veins. I had a friend who had bad piles from time to time, but since she's taken the vitamin E I recommended they are no longer troublesome.'

'Incidentally, to get back to your favourite subject, vitamin E with Kelp does help one to slim. It doesn't peel great tons off you so that you can call it a slimming cure, but the improvement to the circulation combined with the iodine in Kelp does, in a great number of cases, make people much slimmer and keeps them slim once they have got the surplus fat off.'

'I shall certainly take a note of that,' Tana laughed.

'And you feel so well at the same time,' I went on. 'Lastly, Tana, I must tell you, the only snag about vitamin E is that it's rather expensive. But, personally, I would rather give up more expensive face creams and know that by taking vitamin E I should be immensely better-looking than anything the external use of a cream could do for me.'

'How expensive is it?' Tana asked.

'Well, 100 capsules from Healthcrafts, which are the ones I take, cost a guinea,' I said. 'These last me ten days but, really, it isn't very much. I am always amused by women who spend an enormous amount on their clothes, who think nothing of having lunch in a restaurant, and yet complain if you ask them to pay for vitamins – which are the source of life, sex and beauty – that it is too much! What you have got to make up your mind about is which is more important; health and happiness or money in the bank.'

'It may not be in the bank,' Tana said with a smile.

'Well, then I think of the old charwoman who told me that she worked at one of the Ministries, scrubbing the floors,' I said. 'She came into Vitality Fare, a health shop which I was opening at Thayer Street in London. She picked up a packet of Gev-E-Tabs, which contain vitamin E, and said: 'I couldn't work without these. They're worth every penny of what they cost – and a good deal more! She pushed them into her bag and went off to scrub floors. I knew then that I had met a really sensible woman with a proper sense of values!'

CHAPTER VI

Beauty Vitamins

Tana arrived looking very businesslike with a note-book and biro.

'I must take notes,' she said. 'I keep forgetting what you have told me.'

'It's a good idea,' I said. 'Otherwise you will always be telephoning me!'

'I'll try not to be a nuisance,' Tana promised. 'We finished yesterday with you telling me women must be attractive. What other vitamins do I take to help me achieve this?'

'Well, before I go any further,' I said, 'I'm going to tell you what I think is absolutely essential, and that is, anyone who starts to take vitamins should take a foundation capsule. If you take single vitamins, they may be what you need but you may also be deficient in a vitamin of which you have never heard, or one which should balance those you are taking.'

'What do you recommend, then?' Tana asked. 'I believe there are quite a lot of multi vitamin formulas on the market.'

'I take, myself, Gev-E-Tabs made by Healthcrafts,' I replied. 'These contain in one capsule all the vitamins which are thought to be required by the average man or woman during the day. They also contain minerals, which are very important but which are difficult to get singly.'

'Gev-E-Tabs are sold, particularly, for the mature man or woman, but I find them so wonderful that I recommend them to people of all ages. There is a milder capsule made by Healthcrafts, which is called 'Vitamin Mineral', which is extremely useful for children and does often have an excellent effect on older people.' I find, however, that Gev-E-Tabs suit me, suit my Mother and most of my family.'

'What do Gev-E-Tabs contain?' Tana asked.

'Here is the formula,' I said, 'and I give it because I do want people to see how many vitamins and minerals are necessary to us every day. People are always saying to me: 'If I take vitamin B, will it matter if I also take Bio-Strath, or vitamin A, or anything else?' The Answer is: No – take the lot; you can't eat too many vitamins.'

FORMULA

Vitamin E	80 i.u.
Wheat Germ Oil	500 mg.
Vitamin A	15,000 i.u.
Carotene	0.688 mg.
Vitamin D2	400 i.u.
Vitamin B1	6 mg.
Vitamin B2	4 mg.
Vitamin B6	1.0 mg.
Vitamin B12	2 mcg.
Nicotinamide	40.0 mg.
Biotin	1.0 mcg.
Pantothenic Acid	10.0 mg.
Choline	10.0 mg.
Inositol	2.0 mg.

Vitamin C	80.0 mg.
Iron	14.9 mg.
Copper	0.4 mg.
Calcium	28 mg.
Phosphorus	21.6 mg.
Iodine	0.0076 mg.
Magnesium	1 mg.
Potassium	1 mg.
Manganese	0.01 mg.
Zinc	0.1 mg.
Molybdenum	0.1 mg.

'Well, having got my foundation vitamin, what do I do next?' Tana asked.

'I'm not going to give you a whole treatise on vitamins; what they mean; the use of them; and what food one finds them in,' I said. 'To begin with, it's rather boring because you have read it so often before. Secondly, I have already written it down in a book called, *'Vitamins for Vitality'*, which is very instructive. But, we are concerned at the moment with making you beautiful and so I want to concentrate on the vitamins which are essential for youth and beauty.'

'We've already spoken about vitamin B and we have chosen your foundation vitamin capsule. Now, I have discovered recently that people have under-estimated vitamin A, and it is, I believe, one of the main vitamins which affect one's looks. Minor deficiencies of vitamin A are so common that almost everyone you speak to has them without realising it.'

'A very slight deficiency of vitamin A impairs vision.

Both day and night vision requires vitamin A, but night vision depends entirely on the vitamin A mechanism. Therefore, a very small deficiency of vitamin A causes difficulty in seeing in the dark. During the war, when I was Welfare Officer to the Services in Bedfordshire, I looked after over 10,000 R.A.F. personnel and as most of them flew on very secret, very important missions involving night-flying, you can imagine that we talked a great deal about eyesight.'

'Yes, I remember something about that,' Tana said. 'Didn't the pilots eat carrots?'

'Carrots were recommended for pilots who were doing night sorties,' I replied. 'But I only wish that we had known, then, as much about the wonderful, natural vitamins as we do now. You test your vitamin A accuracy any time you drive at night.'

'How do I do that?' Tana asked.

'The lights of oncoming cars,' I told her, 'destroy vitamin A in your eyes. If you have plenty of the vitamin you will see again almost immediately; if you are blinded and it takes some time for you to be able to see again, then you can gauge the severity of your deficiency by the time it takes you to see. Tests have shown that persons have car accidents at night are often terribly deficient in this vitamin.'

'It's rather frightening, isn't it?' Tana said. 'You may have a terrible accident, not because you are driving badly but simply because you are deficient in a vitamin.'

'I can never understand,' I said, 'why the Police and the Minister of Transport do not realise this. It would save so many people's live and so many from being injured for life.'

'The next thing is, you can test yourself by seeing if you experience eye fatigue after you have been watching television. Also, people who are very deficient in vitamin A will suffer pain in their eyes after working at a desk all day. They get headaches and a certain type of nervousness comes entirely from lack of vitamin A.'

'I've sometimes felt my eyes ached after reading late a night,' Tana said.

'Typists and book-keepers, who face the glare of a strong light on white paper, frequently suffer from eye strain,' I said, 'and rush to fit themselves out with spectacles. And the sad thing is, that if they had a diet rich in vitamin A, or took vitamin A tablets, they would find it quite unnecessary to have glasses which, however much people may pretend, are not becoming to a woman.'

'I agree with you,' Tana said, 'and I was going to speak to you about that because I'm terrified that I may have to wear glasses. I think they are definitely ageing.'

'Well, try to gauge your need for vitamin A,' I said. 'We all know that people who ski have to wear dark glasses because there is no glare so destructive of vitamin A as sunlight on snow. But, as a general rule, I think it is a mistake to wear dark glasses in sunlight. I think your eyes should learn to stand up to it and, if they're strong enough, they will.'

'If you are deficient of this Vitamin for a long time, does it really damage the eyes?' Tana said.

'If you really neglect the eyes too long, they become so sensitive that it is difficult to restore them to perfect

75

health again,' I replied. 'Poor families in New York have been found to have corneal ulcers in their eyes which are the same as those which occur in India and China. These are entirely due to malnutrition and, in many cases, I am told, the children have had their eyesight completely restored to health when they are given proper food and plenty of vitamin A.'

'What very few people realise is that office girls, who develop pimples on their skins from working under fluorescent lights, are in need of vitamin A. And, what most women should remember is, that without enough vitamin A their hair becomes dry; it lacks gloss and has that dead, brittle look which is so unbecoming.'

'I was going to ask you which vitamins helped the hair,' Tana said.

'Vitamin A is essential,' I answered. 'And I'll tell you something very interesting. The other day I noticed that a young man was suffering from very bad dandruff. It was not only on his coat collar but I could see it on his hair. Plucking up my courage, I said to him:

''You know, if you took vitamin A, your dandruff would disappear.''

'I could see by his face that he didn't believe me but, rather grudgingly, he agreed to try. I saw him a week later – his hair looked sleek and glossy and there wasn't one trace of dandruff.'

'How extraordinary!' Tana said. 'Was he grateful?'

'I think he'll never be without vitamin A again,' I said with a smile. 'But, vitamin A is not only important externally. A deficiency of this vitamin means abnormalities occur in the tissues which we call mucous membranes. Without vitamin A a person will have sore throat, stuffed-up nose, bad sinuses, aching ears and tell me that they continually suffer from catarrh.'

'When the diet is adequate in vitamin A, these membranes continually secrete a liquid, or mucous, which covers the cells and prevents bacteria from reaching them. Nothing is more unbecoming than sinus trouble!'

'I quite agree with you,' Tana said. 'I have an aunt with sinus trouble; her eyes swell up and she feels awful.'

'Tell her about vitamin A,' I said. 'And tell her, too, not to drink milk.'

'I shall certainly remember that,' Tana said. 'But, I meant to ask you, how soon will vitamin A help the eyes?'

'Research in America,' I said, 'has shown that improvement in mild eye symptoms has occurred in as little as one hour after five 50,000 or 100,000 units of vitamin A have been given. On the other hand, when the deficiency is very bad and the vitamin dose is too small, normal vision may not be recovered for weeks, or even months.'

'How much is the right dose?' Tana asked. 'I thought vitamin A was one of the things of which one could take too much.'

'Vitamin A is one of the bogey-bogeys of the doctors,' I said. 'Toxicity to massive doses has been reported where halibut liver oil has been taken in huge tablespoonsful rather than by drops. But, physicians have frequently recommended curative doses of 200,000 units daily for months, and children have been given 300,000 units daily, for long periods, without apparent harm.'

'Even if a toxic dose has been taken, the damage can be prevented or corrected by an increased intake of vitamin C. Personally, I think that 50,000 units per day, in other words two capsules of the vitamin A which I take, is quite enough for the average person. If you have trouble with your eyes you can always increase it.'

'The Council of Pharmacy and Chemistry of the American Association has approved 25,000 units three times daily for prolonged and chronic deficiency; and 25,000 units twice daily for general treatment. They are convinced that doses of vitamin A are more effective when taken as small amounts twice or three times daily, than all at one time.'

'And, I must tell you, that the addition of vitamin E has been found to double the curative effect of vitamin A.'

'I have found that vitamin A helps people with hay fever and any form of congestion of the nose. Incidentally, vitamin A is essential for sexual virility in a man.'

Tana marked 'Vitamin A' in large letters on the note book.

'And while we are still talking about vitamins,' I went on, 'I want to tell you about a new vitamin – new to me, that is – that I have only just found is so important in being young and beautiful. It has been assumed, in the past, that we got enough vitamin B6 from our food but, recently, as with so many other vitamins, the food has not been adequate and we have found very serious deficiencies. In fact, it is only recently that vitamin B6 deficiencies have been produced in human beings.'

'Hospital patients given an adequate diet, except for

vitamin B6, have developed mental depression, sore lips and tongues and, in time, insomnia, nervousness, dizziness and nausia. What is more extraordinary, is that a deficiency of vitamin B6 can produce eczema.'

'And is, therefore, necessary to our skin,' Tana said.

'Exactly!' I agreed. 'Vitamin B6 is known to be part of the enzymes necessary for the utilisation of both fat and protein, and it has been suggested that the eczema appears because the oil glands of the skin cannot function normally without the vitamin.'

'I'm always meeting people with some form of eczema,' Tana said.

'So am I,' I replied. 'And this will bring them new hope. Also, many animals which have been deprived of vitamin B6, have not only developed, eczema, but extreme irritability, insomnia and nervousness and they have often had convulsions, not unlike epilepsy.'

'But, why did no-one know about it before?' Tana asked.

'We are always discovering new things about the human frame,' I answered. 'But, while we are discovering what we need, the food we eat is getting worse and worse and deficiencies are all the more likely. A doctor in America had a group of patients who were given all the other B vitamins but still complained of weakness, excitability, insomnia, extreme nervousness and difficulty in walking. The moment he gave them vitamin B6, their strength increased, they slept soundly and walked miles a day without any trouble.'

'I shall certainly buy myself plenty of B6,' Tana said, 'and I shall recommend it to my cousin, Margaret, who has suffered from eczema for years.'

'Eczema is one of the most difficult things to cure,' I said, 'but I have heard of the most amazing results with the use of vitamin B6 on, not only children, but older people. I heard one story of a child who had had a tick for years and in two days the tick stopped and, on a diet adequate in B6, has never returned.'

'Then, surely, we ought to be told more about this?' Tana insisted.

'I'm telling you now,' I replied. 'But, I assure you that a great many people will tell you I'm wrong; that vitamins are not important and that we get all we need in our food. All I can answer to that is that in one of the mental hospitals in South America, every incoming patient is made to eat a completely adequate diet, containing all the vitamins, for two months before being taken into the general ward. During this time, a very great percentage of patients recovered completely and are sent home as they are no longer in need of mental health treatment.'

'And, what about the patients in this country?' Tana asked.

'When I go round a mental hospital,' I said, 'I always long to ask them to experiment by giving the patients natural vitamins and food containing a lot of protein. I am sure that a large number of those unhappy, miserable people – who are often just bodies more than human beings – would become alive again.'

'Something ought to be done about them,' Tana sighed.

'I feel mental patients are too often treated as hopeless cases too quickly,' I said. 'They are certainly given better surroundings than used to be the case but the attitude of 'She's mad and nothing can be done about it!' is still far too prevalent. People become mental from the very small maladjustment in their mind. Thyroid is one essential to sanity which is often overlooked. But I mustn't diverge from the subject. We were talking about your eyes. While vitamin A is tremendously important, so is vitamin B2. Animals, such as dogs, ducks, rats, chickens, monkeys, geese, and even fish, when put on diets lacking in vitamin B2, have developed cataract. If the vitamin is given early enough the cataract disappears. If, however, the deficiency is allowed to continue, blindness is inevitable.'

'Apart from aching of the eyes, it is very easy to see the symptoms of vitamin B2 deficiency. The most usual sign is a megenta or purplish tongue, which is the result of stagnant blood being held in the taste buds. Changes in the lips, however, occur earlier; lines or wrinkles may be seen or the lips become crinkled and rough. Tiny flakes of skin may peel from them. Women can see these symptoms just by looking in their mirrors.'

Tana took her vanity case out of her bag, looked in the mirror at her smooth, unwrinkled mouth and gave a sigh of relief.

'You are all right at the moment,' I smiled, 'but I expect you've seen people with their mouths splitting or cracked at the corners. These cracks do not heal easily and break open, and although they do not bleed, they become very sore. If the deficiency continues wrinkles appear, radiating from the mouth, which makes some people appear almost as if they were whistling. You know how ugly these wrinkles are and I've often seen women with their lipstick moving from their lips up into the wrinkles above and below it.'

'What is more frightening is that if the deficiency is very bad, the upper lip can practically disappear. You often see the disappearance of an upper lip in very elderly people.'

'Yes, I've often seen that,' Tana said, 'and wondered why.'

'Lack of vitamin B2,' I said. 'Another thing is, of course, that lack of this vitamin makes our eyes very sensitive to light. Don't you know the sort of person who always feels more comfortable wearing dark glasses and who keeps getting nearer and nearer to the light when he wants to read? And, I've known older people whose eyes water or the lids feel as if a grain of sand was underneath them.'

'This happened to a friend of mine and she told me that she had been to two oculists and they both tested her sight and said there was nothing wrong.'

'My eyes feel gritty', she kept saying to me. I gave her vitamin B2 and within twenty-four hours she rang up and told me the feeling had gone.'

'Why do some people have bloodshot eyes?' Tana asked.

'Because they are lacking in vitamin B2,' I replied. 'After these blood vessels have formed, the blood will drain from them when they take enough vitamin B2, but the blood vessels will remain and blood can quickly enter them again whenever the deficiency occurs. A person whose eyes have once been bloodshot often will have quick recurrences whenever their intake of vitamin B2 is deficient.'

'And what about people who have veins on their faces?' Tana asked. 'I've always been afraid of having them.'

'It is a condition similar to bloodshot eyes,' I replied. 'Tiny blood vessels are formed on the outer layer of the skins which normally would not contain blood vessels. They give the cheeks a high colour and people say how well you look; but this abnormal colouring, which you often see in alcoholics, is really a vitamin deficiency. It will disappear when the person eats the right thing and adds vitamins to their food.'

'I'm only so sorry for the poor things who don't know all this,' Tana said.

'That is why I say that the work I am doing now is a Crusade,' I answered. 'It helps people, not only in their looks, but in their character, in their happiness and in the length of their life.'

'In the meantime, they suffer!' Tana said.

'That's the tragedy!' I said. 'I've known old ladies in the old people's homes who have been able to sew again after they have been given the right amount of vitamins. I know one old woman who wasn't able to watch the television. She used to sit in the room asking the others to tell her what was happening and being, I suspect, a regular nuisance. Only a week or so after she had been given a balanced vitamin diet, and vitamin B2, she was able to watch the programmes. Her delight was pathetic.'

'So, watch your skin. Watch for those little, tiny veins which are a sure sign that something is wrong. One of the worst cases of vitamin B2 deficiency that I've ever seen was in a woman who kept telling me that she had always had apple cheeks and that they ran in her family.'

'Any more vitamins?' Tana asked.

'There are dozens of them,' I replied, 'but I'm just going to pick out what I consider are the most important for you. Don't forget, this is 'The Youth Secret'. I'm not prepared, in this book at any rate, to try and do anything except help you to preserve a radiant youth.'

'Well, what else then?' Tana asked impatiently.

'Vitamin C, of course,' I said. 'No-one can be beautiful if they haven't got enough vitamin C – and no-one can remain young without it, either!'

'One function of vitamin C is to form and maintain collagen, which holds together every cell in your body. Normal blood vessels are amazingly elastic, like rubber bands, but a partial lack of vitamin C causes damage in all the blood vessel walls. When a deficiency exists, the capillary walls break down and the blood is freed into the tissues. These tiny haemorrhages, which cause pain, are spoken of as rheumatism. When adequate vitamin C is added to the diet, however, the capillary walls become strong within twenty-four hours.'

'As quickly as that!' Tana exclaimed. 'I'm always amazed at how swiftly vitamins work.'

'When vitamin C is inadequate the foundation of the bone partially breaks down,' I went on, 'minerals are lost, bones become brittle, lack elasticity and strength, and break easily. Vitamin C is essential to every part of your body.'

'Is this a new vitamin?' Tana asked.

'No, an old one,' I answered. 'During the First World

War it was noticed that wounds healed slowly, or failed to heal, unless fresh fruit was eaten. Experiments proved that the speed of healing and the strength of scar tissue are directly proportional to the vitamin C intake. Anyone who has a scar, a wound, or who is going to have an operation, should take very large amounts of vitamin C, both before and during their time in hospital. Vitamin C, of course, is particularly important to the healing of broken bones.'

'But to get back to your eyes, Tana. Experimental cataracts have been produced by restricting the vitamin C intake. Another thing! What would you say, if I suggested to you that you had scurvy?'

'I should think you were mad!' Tana answered.

'Yet, a doctor at Colombia University pointed out years ago that many signs considered typical of old age, are actually symptoms of scurvy – wrinkles; loss of the elasticity of the skin; loss of teeth; brittleness of bones. He said, all these were really just lack of vitamin C.'

'That means that vitamin C is terribly important if we want to remain young,' Tana said.

'Of course, it is!'

'But, surely, we get enough in fruit?'

'Do you eat a lot of fruit?' I said. 'I find people eat very little fruit in this country, and although most nutritionists recommend fresh orange juice, I don't. I've found that the orange is very inclined to give people eczema; that it's far too strong for the average stomach; and orange juice taken in large quantities does not produce, as people expect, a good skin. If you don't believe me, look at the girls in Canada and America, who very seldom have the clear, almost transparent skin of English women.'

'Do you think their bad complexions are due to all the fruit juice they drink?' Tana asked.

'I think so,' I replied, 'but the women who scream for their orange juice will never believe me. I'm against great dollops of fruit juice of any sort taken at all times of the day. And, I'll tell you one thing, girls who have trouble at period time should never drink or eat fruit either just before the period or during it. It does, in many cases, cause pain.'

'But, I thought orange juice was so good for you,' Tana argued.

'Orange juice averages 130 milligrams of vitamin C,' I said. 'At the same time, if it is too strong for you to digest it's not doing you any good. And, as for the synthetic orange juice which is sold; it is one of the most wicked confidence tricks which the poor, long-suffering public has to put up with. In nearly every case, when investigated, those soft drinks have never seen an orange, or any other fruit. The bottle is made up of chemical flavours, many of which are quite dangerous.'

'Then, what should we do?' Tana asked.

'Eat plenty of green vegetables, to start with,' I said. 'Tomatoes and cabbage average quite a number of milligrams; Brussel sprouts and broccoli are very good sources. But, to be quite certain you are on the right side I advise taking tablets of Acerosa made from Acerola berries, a wonderful source of vitamin C which was discovered in the Caribbean. I find them delicious, and children like sucking them, too.'

'Don't worry that you may take too much vitamin C. I knew one of the Research Chemists who experimented which vitamin C on a great number of school children and he said that in every case where too much was taken, it was eliminated in the urine without any trouble at all. And, don't forget, Tana, if you start bruising you know at once that you are deficient in vitamin C.'

'A friend of mine said she found it brought down a high temperature,' Tana said.

'It has been shown to do that and it does help prevent fatigue. Soldiers who took part in an experiment when they were given plenty of vitamin C, found that they could walk further and carry heavier equipment than their comrades who had not taken the vitamin. Children, of course, can get vitamin C in blackcurrant juice, but do be careful which sort you buy. One of the most advertised in this country contains white sugar.'

'I am also a great believer in Rose Hip Syrup. You can make your own if you are feeling energetic. The Women's Institute have a very good recipe. I take Rose Hip Syrup when I am feeling tired; when I think I am beginning a cold; and, always, if I have a sore throat.'

I looked at the clock!

'What a séance!' I exclaimed. 'I'm sure you are exhausted. We ought to take some Vitamin C right away.'

'I would rather have some of your delicious comb honey,' Tana replied, 'and it will be just as good at making me feel gay and energetic.'

She looked at my face and laughed.

'You see, I haven't forgotten the first lessons you gave me. Tea time is honey time!'

CHAPTER VII

The good Temper Formula

'Barbara, I've got a problem for you!' Tana exclaimed as she entered the drawing-room. She was looking slimmer and I knew she had given up white sugar since our talks. It had fined her face and she really looked ten years younger than she had a month earlier.

'Another!' I groaned, pointing to a huge pile of letters which I had just opened. I answer problems in the magazine, 'Here's Health', and sometimes I think I shall never finish one batch before another lot arrives.

'I've just been talking to Mildred,' Tana said. 'And what do you think she told me?'

'I've no idea,' I murmured, leaving my desk and sitting down on the sofa in front of the fire.

'She says,' Tana answered dramatically, 'that she is so disagreeable that her husband is threatening to leave her!'

'But, that's ridiculous!' I exclaimed. 'Dick adores Mildred.'

'He used to,' Tana said, 'but I've noticed she has gone to pieces a bit lately and become terribly edgy. She snaps his head off at the slightest thing.'

I have known Mildred for years. She is the sort of person who runs the local W.V.S., organises bazaars and is indispensible at Election time. She has a charming husband, two teenage sons and a very comfortable house. She and her husband have been through financial difficulties in the past but now they are financially well-off and Mildred has help with the housework. Why, then, should she be disagreeable?

'I told her you would help her,' Tana was saying.

'Of course, I'll try,' I said.

'I knew you would!' Tana exclaimed. 'So I've brought Mildred with me. She is outside in the car.'

'Then ask her to come in,' I said, jumping up. 'How silly of you to leave her outside!'

'She is feeling shy,' Tana said. 'But, do you mind if I listen to you both? I feel it might help me. Mildred was at school with me and we are practically the same age.'

'You can stay if Mildred doesn't mind,' I replied. 'But ask her first.'

Apparently Mildred didn't mind an audience because they came back into the room together.

'Tana has told you my problem,' Mildred said after we had greeted each other. 'I'm so ashamed of myself, I really am, but I just can't help being so cross and irritable. I love Dick but every evening when he comes home from the office, we seem to have a row and I know it's my fault!'

She was near to tears and Tana pressed her hand.

'I take vitamins,' Mildred went on, 'all the ones you recommend – but even they don't help.'

'How much bonemeal do you take?' I asked.

'Bonemeal?' she queried. 'Well, actually, none. I know it's good for teeth, but as I've lost mine I thought there was no need for me to take it any more.'

'But one of the most important things in our diet as we grow older is calcium,' I said. 'And I suspect, Mildred, that is the whole trouble. When we are emotionally upset, disagreeable or angry, we use up calcium in our bodies. This must be replaced, otherwise we become badly deficient.'

'Could that be making me so irritable?' Mildred asked.

'Of course it could,' I replied. 'In fact, when I feel 'on edge' I always take extra bonemeal, just as I take it when I can't sleep. I am convinced that everyone needs lots more calcium.'

Mildred looked unconvinced and I went on:

'Dr. Clive McCay, of Cornell University, published a report proving that women from the age of fifty-two need a gram of calcium a day if they want to keep their bones hard and their nerves healthy.'

'I shall be fifty-one next May,' Mildred murmured.

'Then start at once,' I begged her. 'Dr. McCay, in his experiments with animals, found that young animals could store about 78 to 88 per cent of the calcium they are. But animals old enough to compare with human beings of fifty, could not even maintain what calcium they had in their bodies, let alone store more.'

'I thought I read somewhere that you could take too much calcium and it would cause hardening of the arteries,' Mildred said.

'That's nonsense!' I replied. 'Dr. McCay, who is one of America's leading authorities on nutrition, has answered that question. He says: 'In the course of two decades of research with rats we have seen groups, at the time of death, with heavily calcified arteries and kidneys. This calcification of soft tissues was due to unknown variables in the diet and could never be related to dietary calcium.'

'How much should I take?' Mildred asked.

'I take six bonemeal tablets every day,' I answered, 'and I intend to increase the intake every year as I get older. I must tell you about my Mother. Five years ago, when she was eighty-five, she was running downstairs and banged against a square newel at the turn of the staircase. She fractured a rib!'

'At eighty-five!' Mildred exclaimed.

'That's what worried me,' I said. 'Because when people of that age break a bone, it sometimes doesn't heal.'

'What happened?' Mildred asked.

'I rang up my Mother and asked her what she was doing. She said: 'Well, it's very painful but I'm taking bonemeal.' 'How much?' I enquired. 'Twelve a day,' she replied. 'Mummy, you're wonderful!' I exclaimed. And now the fantastic end to the story. My Mother's fractured rib was healed in three weeks. The doctor was astonished; he said he didn't expect a girl of eighteen to heal as quickly as that.'

'I'm not surprised that the doctor was astonished,' Mildred cried. 'It was over six months before my Mother's arm healed when she broke it and she was only sixty-eight.'

'Older people should take a large amount of calcium every day,' I said firmly. 'Bone broth is easy to make and very cheap. A butcher will invariably produce a big bone for nothing, or a few pence, if one asks for it. And there's one thing I want to say very firmly – bonemeal is not a medicine; it is a food. Bonemeal is only whole bones ground up so that we do not have to chew them.'

'Bones were used by man very early in history. Recorders have discovered that he ate fish bones and that when he was unable to chew the bones of the animals he had hunted and killed, he pounded them up so that they could be eaten more easily. How wise primitive man was in his instinct to eat what was best for him, is shown in an analysis of the minerals in a typical sample of bonemeal. This was prepared by the Department of Agriculture in the U.S.A.

	Per Cent		Per Cent
Sodium oxide	.46	Lead oxide	.005
Potassium oxide	.20	Zinc oxide	.018
Calcium oxide	30.52	Chlorine	.22
Magnesium oxide	.73	Phosphoric oxide	22.52
Barium oxide	.001	Buron oxide	trace
Copper oxide	.0005	Fluorine	.043
Iron oxide	.004	Iodine	.00002
Manganese oxide	.0014	Sulphur	.25

'It sounds good!' Mildred exclaimed.
'It is,' I agreed. 'I only wish I had known about bonemeal when I was young. I had constant trouble with my teeth but do you know that now, when I go to the dentist every six months – as every sensible person should do – he just cleans them and sends me away. Also, my sons very, very seldom need a filling.'
'Surely bonemeal is what the authorities should give school children!' Mildred exclaimed.

'Of course, it is,' I replied, 'instead of advocating that the dangerous poison, Sodium Fluoride, should be added to the water supplies! Do you know that Dr. A. Aslander, of the Royal Institute of Technology, Stockholm, experimented with bonemeal in a region where only one child in a thousand was free from dental caries?'

'And what was the result?' Mildred asked.

'A mouthful of perfectly healthy teeth in each case!' I replied.

'Then why doesn't Great Britain follow Sweden?' Mildred asked.

'I was in America the other day,' I replied, 'and there was a cartoon in one of the newspapers showing great mountains of Sodium Fluoride – the residue of an aluminium factory – and a man was saying: 'We must get rid of all this; let's shove it in the water supplies.' It makes me furious to talk about it. So, let us return to bonemeal. When you are sleeping badly, take honey in hot water last thing at night and three or four bonemeal tablets. When you have a headache you will find bonemeal removes it far quicker than those awful headache tablets which are really bad for you.'

'I shall certainly try it,' Mildred said.

'One word of warning,' I continued. 'Calcium needs vitamin D to make it digestible, so before you buy a packet see that the tablet also contains vitamin D. The type I take come from Health-crafts; the tablets also contain Rose Hips and Brewers' Yeast to facilitate complete assimilation. The joy is that it is also very cheap.'

'I'm going to buy some right away,' Mildred cried.

'And don't forget your other vitamins,' I called after her. 'Bonemeal is ideally taken with Gev-E-Tabs, vitamin E and, of course, Bio-Strath.'

'I shall be so good tempered that Dick will fall in love with me all over again,' Mildred cried. 'Thank you, Barbara! I can't tell you how grateful I am.'

She kissed me goodbye and when she had gone I looked at Tana with a twinkle in my eyes.

'Have you learned a lesson from Mildred?' I asked.

'Don't worry about me!' Tana replied. 'I'm going to order a crate of the stuff; and what's more, everyone in my household is going to take it – whether they like it or not!'

'Very wise,' I approved. 'Marriages have broken up before now on nothing more sensational than the lack of a bonemeal tablet!'

CHAPTER VIII

Sleep Well

Tana and I were sitting down in my drawing-room and the door opened and a great friend put her head round the door.

'A little bird called Mildred told me about these beauty sessions,' she said. 'I've come with my special problem!'

'Come in, Claressa,' I said. 'I haven't seen you for ages! What's wrong?'

'I was reading an article of yours last week,' she said, 'and in it you said that sleeping tablets were dangerous. Now, I just don't believe that, and I've come to ask you what you think one should take if one doesn't sleep.'

'Certainly not sleeping tablets,' I replied.

'It's no use, I have to take them!' Claressa said defiantly. 'I can't lie awake hour-after-hour, tossing from side to side and feeling infuriated. Of course, the angrier I get, the less I sleep.'

'And so, your hand goes out and you take one of those horrid little white or yellow capsules,' I said. 'Have you looked at your face lately?'

'Of course,' Claressa replied. 'Why?'

'Have you noticed those dark lines under your eyes; the sharpening of the lines from your nose to your mouth; the way your chin is beginning to sag a little?'

'Oh, that!' she exclaimed. 'Well, I did think I was getting rather peaky; I thought it was just being tired and a bit run-down.'

'You are thirty-nine,' I said reflectively. 'By the time you are forty-five you will look sixty.'

'But, why? Why?' she asked.

'Sleeping tablets produce the mast ghastly lines in a woman's face,' I replied. 'I had a friend who was one of the great beauties of the Twenties. She took to sleeping tablets and her skin gradually lost all its elasticity and nourishing oils. She had lines like an old, old woman by the time she was fifty-five!'

'But everyone takes them sometime in their life,' Claressa protested.

'Eight hundred and fifty million sleeping tablets and tranquillisers were prescribed last year on the National Health alone,' I told her. 'There were also fifty thousand attempted suicides.'

'What has that got to do with it?'

'All sedatives are depressing. Take a sleeping draught and you wake up feeling muzzy, limp and rather under-the-weather. Do this several nights running and you wake up really depressed. The obvious course, the, is to pep yourself up. This stop-go is what has killed many famous film stars!'

'But, one needn't be so exaggerated; it's only occasionally,' Claressa pleaded.

'That's exactly what the L.S.D. and Purple Hearts addicts started by saying. I am absolutely convinced that sedatives and dope eventually destroy, mentally and physically, those who take them.'

'Is that really true?' Claressa asked.

'I had a letter a little while ago,' I told her, 'from a man whose wife had been a brilliant scientist. She had loved her home, her husband and her children, but she got run down, found she was sleeping badly, and started taking sleeping tablets. Her husband told me that she had gone utterly to pieces. She didn't care about her family or anything else. She just drifted through life in a meaningless fog.'

'It's terrifying, but I shan't get like that.'

'Why not?' I asked. 'You think you have so much will power, but already when you don't sleep you can't say, no, to the temptation of a pill. Each time you take one you are weaker, less positive, less in control of yourself and your emotions.'

'What about herbs?' Claressa asked.

'They are better for your health, admittedly, but they have almost the same effect. I've never taken insomnia herbs of any sort without having a hang-over, without feeling low and depressed in the morning. All sedatives and narcotics are the enemies of vitamins – they kill them.'

'But, herbs are healing,' Claressa insisted.

'People think all herbs are good, which is nonsense!' I replied. 'The ancients knew the dangers of narcotic herbs and ascribed their uses to Circe – the evil enchantress. You will remember that Nepanthe, one of her concoctions, caused her victims to lose their memories and make them her slaves.'

'I can see the moral in that story,' Claressa smiled.

'Personally, I think honey is the best sedative in the world,' I said, 'and really is good for your health. Honey has the unique quality of being naturally an energiser and a sedative. It is also nature's most wonderful healer.'

'What do *you* do about insomnia?' Claressa asked. 'Don't tell me you always sleep like a log. You have far too much on your mind.'

'I take honey in hot water or peppermint tea,' I replied, 'and bone-meal tablets which are, of course, calcium with vitamin D. Some-one has said that calcium is as soothing as a mother, as relaxing as a sedative and as life saving as an oxygen tent!'

'Will that really make me sleep?' Claressa asked.

'I think that sleeplessness falls into two main categories,' I said. '*First*, because we are suffering from over-work, sorrow, shock, or just that most beastly of all complaints – worry. *Secondly*, indigestion.'

'I often have indigestion,' Claressa said.

'I expect you have it a great deal more often than you think,' I said. 'But first of all, do try to stop worrying. The whole world is a worrying place, but we've got to live in it and, however strong we may be, we can't alter more than a very small part in which we live ourselves. Worry, however great the cause, does become acute when we're tired, under-nourished and sick; and when we worry we destroy the vitamins in our bodies.'

'So the first thing to do,' Tana interposed, 'is to increase our vitamin intake, both in our food and in our tablets. You see how well I am beginning to understand what you are trying to say, Barbara?'

'I'm very glad,' I said, 'because it's true. And sorrow – something which we all encounter in our lives, sometime or another, depletes our bodies very quickly of theid vitamin content. But, the very worst thing to take

98

if you are unhappy, is a tranquilliser.'

'Tranquillisers, like sleeping pills, merely accentuate what you are feeling already. They give you a short time when you are anaesthetised but, if you take them when you are unhappy, when you wake up you will be still more unhappy – and they have frightening side-effects.'

'What do you mean by that?' Claressa asked.

'I was given a tranquilliser some time ago,' I answered, 'when I had a slipped rib which was very painful. It dulled the pain and I thought it was excellent; I was beginning to recommend it to people, until one day when I was sitting up in bed reading the newspaper and tears suddenly began to pour out of my eyes in a stream. I wasn't unhappy and I wasn't crying but my eyes had lost control. It was a terrifying moment which I shall never forget!'

'You'd better put that tranquillisers, whatever it was, on the list of things we mustn't take,' Tana said.

'All tranquillisers are bad,' I said. 'I wouldn't give them to anyone. After my husband died, I was desperately unhappy; but I didn't feel the shock of his death, which was very sudden, until about six months later. And, then, suddenly, I began to feel so miserable, so nervy, so tearful, that I was frightened of myself. But, you know, when things happen to us, when we are in dire need, we are always helped.'

'How were you helped?' Tana asked softly.

'I have already mentioned Bio-Strath to you,' I said. 'This is what happened about it. A man came to see me from Switzerland. He had come to talk about antifluoridation, on which he was a great expert, and I said to him during the course of the conversation: 'I suppose, coming from Switzerland, you don't know of a new tonic? I feel I need one at the moment.''

'He said: 'As a matter of fact, I do. I know of a very marvellous, herbal tonic called Bio-Strath.'

''What does it do?' I asked.

''It makes all the difference in the world to your life,' he replied.

'Well, to cut a long story short, he sent me a bottle, and, from the moment I took it, I felt so different. I was still unhappy, of course, but I could cope with my own unhappiness and myself. Well, a little while later, he rang me up and said:

''You are so enthusiastic about the Bio-Strath I sent you, I wonder if you'd like to come out to Switzerland and see it being made?'

'I had a week-end free and I said I'd go. I flew to Zurich, where I was met by Mr. Frederick Pestalozzi, who owns Bio-Strath – he is a cousin of Henri Pestalozzi, who started the Orphans' Homes in Switzerland. A small, wiry little man with very blue eyes, seeming full of energetic, vital health, I was astounded to learn, later, that he had suffered from Meniers Disease, which means that you get dizzy, fall down easily and, eventually, go stone deaf. Mr. Pestalozzi took his own Bio-Strath and today I cannot imagine a fitter or more energetic man.'

'We drove up the mountains to a laboratory which overlooked the Lake of Geneva and the snowy peaks of the Jungfrau. From the moment I entered that laboratory,

100

I had a sense of well-being, of cleanliness, of health, and I knew that something exceptional was happening there.'
'I had already learned that Bio-Strath had been invented by Professor Strathmeyer who, in the war, was working as a chemist for the Germans. They had given him the task of making sugar from wood and he had said to himself: 'A live body needs a live medicine; after the war I will make one.' He settled in Switzerland and invented Torula yeast. Today, ninety mountain plants, growing organically, are chopped up like grass mowings and put into huge vats with the Torula yeast. The yeast devours them, or, as they say in Germany, explodes the cell; and after three weeks a dark brown liquid comes from the vats. This is Bio-Strath, a pure, unadulterated, herbal elixir, without the addition of any chemicals.'
'I was so excited by what I saw and what I had already proved to myself, by taking Bio-Strath, that I felt this was something that must be available to to overyone. I went back to England and rang up the Assistant Editor of the 'Daily Mail'.'
'Derrick Ingram is an old friend and I said to him: 'I've found something thrilling! You will remember you wrote about H.3 when Olga Franklin went to Bucharest and discovered our dear friend, Professor Ana Aslan? Well, I've discovered something just as wonderful and you've got to tell you readers about it.'
''All you've got to do is to convince our Science Adviser, Hugh McLeave,' he said. 'He'll come down and see you.'
'Hugh McLeave came to lunch and he wrote a brilliant

101

article in the 'Daily Mail'. And, from that one article, people in Great Britain began to buy Bio-Strath. When you sell an ordinary product people buy it because it's advertised or because they've heard about it and, if it's no good, they finish the bottle or throw it away and never think about it again. But, Bio-Strath went on selling, because people felt so much better; they found it cured so many things in them. So they went back for another bottle, and yet another, and now it is one of the biggest, if not the biggest, single health product on sale in this country.'

'Fred Pestalozzi had to work in his little laboratory day and night. Soon he had to enlarge it and put in a bigger plant. Where I had seen 6,000 bottles a day being filled, he now has a bottler which fills 16,000 at the same time – and still the demand increases.'

'Sir Stanley Matthews, one of our greatest sportsmen, tells me that he takes Bio-Strath every day; and Bio-Strath sales follow wherever I go. Mrs. Indira Gandhi, the President of India, has found it a tremendous help, and surely no woman had a more gigantic task to perform! The Queen of Bhutan, exquisite and lovely, who lives, literally, on what is known as, 'the roof of the world', told me that both she and her husband take it. In Mexico I gave it to a number of people who have all written to me and told me how wonderful they feel after it. A friend in Jamaica has ordered a case to be sent to her by air, every month; in Bangkok and Hong Kong, people have thanked me for bringing Bio-Strath into their lives.'

'Well, what exactly does it do?' Claressa asked.

'I think what it really does is to balance the body,' I said. 'We are all so terribly deficient in so many ways, it is almost impossible to pinpoint them. Bio-Strath is really the Magical Elixir, for which people searched in the Middle Ages. It does restore youth and good health.'
'There is nobody today who doesn't feel tired and weary from the noise and bustle, with the inadequate food, the worry and difficulties. Bio-Strath makes you able to cope with all of these. It doesn't divorce you from the world; it makes you strong enough to face what has to be faced and that's far more important than running away.'
'So, I should take Bio-Strath for insomnia?' Claressa said.
'If you have insomnia, you must feed your nerves with large quantities of vitamins – especially vitamin B – honey, plenty of protein – meat, fish, chickens and eggs – and take lots of exercise in the fresh air. Even if you work in an office you can walk for miles at a week-end or play games, and during the week you can walk at least some of the way to work. Before you set off in the morning, take your Bio-Strath; if you have got to go out in the evening, take it when you get home.'
'How much do I take?' Claressa asked.
'You can read what it says on the bottle,' I answered, 'but, I'll confess to you, that I take a great deal more. I don't believe you can take too much and I know that in my madly busy life, the only way I can get through is by taking Bio-Strath.'
'And, now, to go back to the causes of insomnia, I must speak about indigestion.'

103

'I often have indigestion,' Tana said. 'And, now you talk about it, I believe it does keep me awake a night.'

'People often have indigestion without knowing it,' I said. 'The answer, of course, is to find out what has upset your stomach. Protein digests slowly – some things are slower than others. Veal, for instance, takes longer than lamb. Many things are not easily absorbed and everyone has their individual substances which they find indigestible. I can't eat mushrooms at night, or fruit of any kind; and no green vegetables. I don't, as a rule, get a pain, but I just don't sleep.'

'Cooked cheese is indigestible at night to many people; so is pork and very spicy dishes. Make a list and avoid all these things. I find that I often think, 'It will be all right tonight,' but it never is!'

'And if you do eat them, what do you do?' Claressa asked.

'I take two tablets of Herb Formula D,' I replied, 'and Ver-O-Vine, from Heath and Heather, an entirely herbal preparation containing mistletoe, which will usually settle my stomach if all else fails. Incidentally, I can't sleep if I have anything alcoholic to drink after eight o'clock.'

'Why is that?' Tana asked.

'I think that alcohol gets more difficult to digest as one gets older. The fumes rise into your brain and you find yourself lying awake thinking about things. It's a bore to refuse wines if you go to many dinner parties, but alcohol is another weapon used as an escape route from reality and is dangerous and ineffective. Drinking only accelerates your feelings; if you are unhappy, you will feel more unhappy; if you are worried, you will worry more.'

'One can't help worrying so what can one do for nerves?' Claressa asked.

'Nerves, which are an almost universal modern complaint are mainly the result of wrong feeding,' I answered. 'Take Bio-Strath and you will not have nerves. What is more, you will begin to feel so much younger and so much gayer. I've never met anyone taking Bio-Strath who didn't feel happier; which really means that their body has begun to balance itself.'

'Is it fattening?' Tana asked.

'On the contrary, it's slimming!' I answered. 'I know a man, an ordinary, working man, who took Bio-Strath because he felt so ill. I gave him the first bottle and then he bought himself three bottles because he said it made all the difference to his life, and he lost half-a-stone in a month.'

'Is there anything else I should take?' Claressa asked.

'Well, there has been a great deal of talk about magnesium,' I answered. 'This is a component of chlorophyll and as a mineral it is necessary to the action of thirty eczymes in the body. The best source is green leaves, like potassium, which, however, is easily lost in the cooking water. When animals are deficient in magnesium their hearts usually become abnormal and beat too rapidly and they become nervous and irritable and often have tremors or convulsions. In fact, the animal's behaviour resembles certain types of insanity.'

'We always seem to be getting back to irritability,' Tana said to Claressa with a little sigh.

'Irritability is one of the danger signals which tell us that something is wrong with our bodies,' I answered. 'And the blood of persons suffering from extreme irritability is found to be very low in magnesium. Scientists working on this have found that vitamin B6, of which we have already said quite a lot, helps the utilisation of magnesium, and I believe that magnesium deficiencies may be partly responsible for widespread nervousness and insomnia.'

'How do I take magnesium?' Tana asked.

'In tablet form,' I answered. 'Dolomite tablets are now available at almost every Health Store. I take three a day and I'm quite certain that they have helped me, both to sleep and in other ways as well. Dolomite tablets come from a deeply mined rock in the Dolomites and they contain two minerals – calcium and magnesium. Scientists are beginning, more and more, to realise that magnesium is something which the body requires and I think to be able to take it in tablet form makes it so simlpe.'

'Lastly, while we are still talking about insomnia, I do beg of you not to let the sun go down on your wrath. I know nothing that keeps one awake worse than tossing and turning and going over what one has said to somebody and thinking what one will say to them tomorrow, or the next day, or, perhaps, the letter you will write to them. However difficult it may be, do say you are sorry. What does it matter? One is always sorry if there's been a row, whether one is right or wrong.'

'It's being pretty magnanimous when you know you are in the right!' Claressa said.

'Who is to know, for an absolute surety, whether you are right or wrong? Everybody thinks they are right when they get mixed up in an argument or a quarrel,' I replied. 'And, if you want to sleep well and feel at peace with the world, then you'll make-up any quarrel, however trivial or however big, before you go to bed.'

'I think you are asking rather a lot,' Claressa said.

'I feel that at night we never get things quite into the right proportion,' I said. 'One has a terrible quarrel, we'll say, with one's husband or children over something. Does it really matter, beside the fact that you have spent many years of your life with them and will probably spend many more? Remember that you love them and they love you! Suppose they died during the night, would you ever forgive yourself that they had left you with something ugly and horrible unsettled between you?'

'If you put it like that, the answer, of course, is that nothing matters except them,' Claressa answered.

'Then, make it up,' I said. 'Make it up and sleep peacefully. And, I know it's old-fashioned and out-of-date today, but a prayer before you go to sleep – a prayer not asking for something, but of gratitude for all you've had, for being alive and well and having so much to be thankfull for – is the way to sleep peacefully.'

CHAPTER IX

The Constant Lover

I knew when Tana came into the room, that she had something on her mind. I hadn't seen her for a week and after talking about a lot of unimportant things there was a sudden silence.

'I want to know more about the vitamins which help a man whose sex life is slowing down,' Tana said a little diffidently, not looking at me as she spoke.

I guessed this was a delicate subject where she was concerned, for her husband is older than she is and I had thought for some time that there was a something almost antagonistic between them, as if they were not getting along as well sexually as they had in the past. So, I chose my words rather carefully.

'Some years ago,' I said, 'in a speech I made in Hatfield, I said that young wives couldn't expect to have a virile, exciting husband if they fed him on sandwiches. A man needed meat and two veg. to be a competent lover! The National Newspapers reported this and Giles drew a very funny cartoon which later he signed for me.'

'Oh! I've seen it,' Tana said.

'The truth is that women, especially British women,' I went on, 'still do not realise 'we are what we eat', and have no idea that the average husband is suffering from concealed malnutrition.'

'Oh, really, Barbara, you do exaggerate!' Tana exclaimed.

'It's true, unfortunately,' I replied. 'Think about it. At the beginning of the century, a man was regarded as a strong, passionate creature with whom no attractive woman was safe. In the wealthy classes, girls were chaperoned, hedged around by conventions and subjected to interminable lectures on the virtue of chastity, just because men were so dangerous. And, for the shop girl, the woman servant and the girl working in a factory, her whole existence was subjected to the fact that she must keep men at arm's length or find herself in the ghastly position of being thrown into the street because she was having an unwanted baby.'

'I always thought that was a joke,' Tana said.

'It was no joke to the girls of that period,' I answered. 'The unmarried mother in every class was an outcast and the only future for her was prostitution.'

'Poor things!' Tana said.

'In those days,' I continued, 'for a woman of any age to go to a man's flat, or rooms, was to be damned socially, as no-one would believe, for one moment, that she had not been seduced on arrival.'

'How extraordinary!' Tana exclaimed. 'Is that really true?'

'I've heard my Mother say that certain streets in London were barred to ladies walking alone, or even with a friend of the same sex,' I replied. 'Bond Street was one, while the Burlington Arcade was completely taboo. While in the working classes, the girls who worked for necessity were in continual danger from their employers and other workers of the opposite sex. The history of morality in the mines, the cotton mills and, in fact, in-

109

dustry as a whole, is terrifying to read.'

'Yes, I have seen that in some books of the period,' Tana said.

'Women's partial emancipation,' I went on, 'came with World War I. But, what altered the whole relationship between the sexes was the millions of men killed in action and the tremendous surplus of women – I think there were two million in 1919! More important still, the men returning to civilian life were tired and nervous after the horror and privation of the trenches. In fact, the swash-buckling, primitive, all-conquering male was already changing into the milk-and-water variety of modern times.'

'Isn't that rather unkind?' Tana asked.

'I'm afraid,' L replied, 'that the age of mechanical progress has been hard both on men and women. Not only has the human body had to adjust itself to travelling at 600 miles an hour, to incessant noise, to suffocatingly packed crowds, to airless, overcrowded places of work and sleep, to a ceaseless round of hustle, bustle, rush and dash, but the mind has also to work under these conditions.'

'Yes, that's true,' Tana said. 'When one is tired in one's mind, it's difficult to feel sexy.'

'Mankind is incredibly adaptable,' I said, 'but in the last twenty years everything has accelerated until it is hardly believable that he can survive the conditions that he, himself, has created. And, what is more, the reformation of modern life stifles the energy and enterprise by its machine-like monotony and regularity. That is something which also affects sex.'

'How?' Tana asked.

'Men and women get up, eat, work and play and go to bed, at precisely the same time every week-day,' I told her, 'carry on this routine even at week-ends, when they can vary it if they wish.'

'I know some friends who are always called at 7.30 o'clock every day of the week,' Tana said.

'How ridiculous!' I exclaimed. 'And what is the result? It is that men, particularly, are paying the price of financial prosperity by a poverty of sexual capacity.'

'I'm afraid that's true,' Tana said, rather wistfully.

'Sex, for a man,' I continued, 'is something which requires both stimulus and health. Given a pleasurable job he likes, no unusual strain or worry, and good food, a man is what he is created to be – a powerfully sexed creature. But, give him a life of constant anxiety, force him to over-tire his body to the point of exhaustion and feed him with food that has no real sustinence in it, then a man loses his sexual impetus and gradually becomes what he calls 'impotent'.'

'If he mentions it at all,' Tana said. 'You know how embarrassed they are about it.'

'Of course, they're embarrassed,' I replied. 'But, actually, it is not impotency; it is nothing of the sort! It's just a natural withdrawal of desire because the man is starved of the vital substances which make any human being function normally to procreate the species. But, for many husbands and wives, it is a tragedy which should never, and need never, have happened.'

'That's true,' Tana said. 'I have a friend who has left her husband simply because he never seems to desire her as he used to do.'

'And was he a man who worked hard?'

'Oh, very hard!' she said. 'He had to travel to America a lot and nothing is more tiring than that journey backwards and forwards across the Atlantic. But, she is a very passionate person and she just couldn't stand him coming back and being nice to her but not making love.'

'I get letters like that,' I said. 'I had a letter last week in which the man said: 'For some years, now, I have been unable to make love to my wife. I'm ashamed and humiliated but I'm afraid there's nothing I can do about it.' Do you know, that man was only fifty! And another letter from a man only a little bit older said: 'I'm getting more and more impotent and my wife is fifteen years younger than I am. What can I do?' I've received hundreds of letters like this and in nearly every case I've been able to help these unhappy husbands.'

'You have!' Tana said. 'But, how?'

'It's much more simple than it sounds,' I replied. 'If a man has once been a competent lover, then there's no reason why he should ever stop being one. It is, I agree, a pity that there has ever been a break or a slowing down in his desire, but in ninety-nine cases out of a hundred I can help him back to physical happiness. But, he must build on a foundation of health.'

'You mean that it's diet and the whole way of living, besides just taking the magic pill, vitamin E, or something?' Tana asked.

'That's exactly what I am trying to say,' I said. 'You see, people have got so used to going to the doctor, who gives them a pill – antibiotic, or whatever it is – and they imagine that everything can work that way. Well, we now know, as I have tried to explain to you, that it doesn't. The body has got to work completely as a whole, especially where sex is concerned. It amazes me how a man will speak quite learnedly on stock-breeding, knowing the greatest care is taken in feeding the stallions, the bulls and the boars, but he never applies the same yardstick to himself.'

'No, that's true,' Tana said. 'And, of course, the trouble is that women are very much inclined to put their husbands off by saying. 'Oh, you're so old!' or showing that they're not satisfied when he's made love to them.'

'Women are such fools,' I said. 'The real Elixir of Youth is love. A woman who is made love to sexually, who responds, and who is happy, is keeping herself young. Do you know what in the act of love we use every muscle in our body? There is no exercise to equal it.'

'Women don't realise this,' Tana murmured.

'I'm absolutely convinced,' I said, 'that it is the woman's fault, in ninety-nine cases out of a hundred, that a marriage begins to break down sexually. I had a letter from a woman the other day who said: 'My husband is no longer making love to me and I've given him three months in which to do it, otherwise I'm going to leave him.' I wrote back and said – 'A man has to feel desire before he can perform the sexual act, and if he isn't attracted by his wife then, obviously, it's not his fault, but hers. And,' I continued, 'I can imagine nothing more likely to put a man off than being given a time

113

limit. I think that his so-called impotency is your fault in that you have not fed him properly and have lost your attractiveness'.'

'Can a man make love too much in his youth?' Tana asked.

'No!' I said positively. 'This is a question I'm often asked. Some people believe a man can do too much at one period of his life so that he hasn't any vigour left at another. The truth is, the more a man does it the more he can. But, he must go on making love. If any of us cease to use one limb of our bodies, it withers and can no longer function.'

'But, what must a man eat to be virile?' Tana asked.

'First,' I said, 'I am strongly in favour of meat eating for those who want to remain sexually potent in their old age. Every nation in the world has centuries' old diets for potency and, without exception, they all include meat. This also means venison and hares. Protein is the main food a man requires. Dieticians say that the requirement of an average man is 70 grams a day and, to show you what this means, here's a chart:

			Grams of Protein
Beef	average helping		17
Chicken (not caponised)	,,	,,	17
Liver	,,	,,	19
Steak	,,	,,	21
Egg	,,	,,	6
Salmon	,,	,,	22
Soya Flour	1 cupful		37
Wheat Germ	2 cupsful		24

'I'd no idea that soya flour was so high in protein,' Tana said.

'It's a very useful, cheap food for people who can't afford an enormous amount of beef,' I said. 'It's not very nice, but you can put it into sauces, gravies and other forms of cooking so that you don't notice it, and it does do you good. Of course, now we have come back to what I was telling you before; the next important food for sex is vitamin E. So, here we have the crux of the problem. Because food today has had so much of its goodness destroyed, a man must supplement his intake with natural vitamins which should be on his plate but which are not.'

'But how can one make a man take them?' Tana asked.

'Men hate fussing over their health,' I agreed, 'but what I am suggesting is not medicine but food. Here is my list to cure and prevent sexual fatigue and make a man the strong lover he was intended to be by nature:

Protein – as much as he can eat of meat, fish, eggs and cheese (unprocessed).

Fruit and vegetables – but not in abnormal amounts; just what he fancies.

Honey in large quantities.

Gev-e-tabs, 2 every day.

Vitamin E, 10 every day.

Wheat Germ Oil, 4 every day.

Vitamin A, 4 every day.

Bonemeal, 4 every day.

Liver-Plus, 6 every day.

Celaton CH3 Plus. A fabulous sex virility pill.*

Bio-Strath Elixir, 2 desert spoonsful before breakfast and before lunch.

* Note Celaton CH3 Plus can only be bought direct from Biocosmetics see page 149.

Celaton CH3 Plus The amazing combination of H3 and Celaton Biostimulins results in a resurgence of sexual interest and vitality. Marvellously effective.

Pumpkin Seeds – the way these seeds keep a man sexually potent until he reaches a great age is well known in Bulgaria. They also prevent prostate gland.

Forbidden
White bread and very little of any other sort.
White sugar.
Milk.
Coffee.
Smoking.
Beer.
And, most important, Whisky.
If a man feels he must drink spirits, then Brandy is the best of them. Light wines, especially white, are often helpful.

'It seems rather a lot of vitamins,' Tana said pensively.
'I find that most men take them gladly when they realise it is really going to help them,' I said. 'Nothing is more degrading and more humuliating for a man than to feel that he is no longer 'a man'.'
'I agree there,' Tana said with feeling.
'There are, of course, many new rejuvenation treatments, much used on the Continent, which are now easily obtainable in this country,' I continued. 'I have seen tremendous results in men after having H.3 injections, and Celaton CH3 Plus Tablets which are fantastic for virility, are obtainable from Biocosmetics.
'Professor Ana Aslan is a great friend of mine. I met her

when she first came here from Bucharest to lecture on her wonderful discovery. She has grown hair on bald heads; she has made men of 100 do hand-stands; and, most of all, she has given back sexual potency to hundreds and thousands of men who thought they were past 'all that sort of thing'.'

'How wonderful!' Tana said.

'Yes, but the average man,' I said, 'suffering from sexual fatigue, doesn't need anything so drastic. He just wants feeding! It's up to those lazy wives, who think that a man can be virile on a cereal breakfast, a sandwich lunch and a bit of 'made-overs' for dinner.'

'I think, sometimes, women hate their husbands and really try to destroy them. My doctor wrote a book called, 'How to Murder your Husband'; which was nothing more dramatic than nagging and feeding him badly. I am horrified at what men have to put up with, and I'm sure it's because they are so badly fed that they are too exhausted to go home and give their wives a good beating and make them cook a decent dinner for them!'

'You'll be popular with the women!' Tana laughed.

'I don't care,' I answered. 'Every woman should learn to be a cook or be ashamed to be called a woman; and every woman who loves her family should learn a little about diet and the dangers of modern food.'

'And, let us make it quite clear, the stimulus for sex comes from the attraction of a woman and the modern wife should take the trouble to learn that the act of sex requires skill, experience and, above all, love, to make it the ecstasy and glory it was meant to be.'

'You think it's all up to us?' Tana said, reflectively.

'Of course, it is,' I answered. 'A man is a hunter by nature. If you keep a man captive by marrying him, you've got to go on stimulating him; you've got to go on exciting him. As one doctor said to me: 'The women who come to see me and complain about their husbands being inadequate are always the ones who grease their faces, talk about the price of potatoes, then get into bed and expect to be made love to!'

Desire is engendered nowadays, not only by the mere sight of a woman, but because she learns to be attractive, to stimulate the imagination, to arouse desire because she, herself, is desirable. In every marriage where the woman complains that her husband is 'no good' I would ask her: 'Are you the cause of it?' If a man starts by being attracted by a woman she can, if she is clever, and if she really goes out of her way to make herself desirable, keep that attraction alive.'

'How?' Tana asked. 'What should a woman do?'

'Oh, I don't mean that she has got to sit about all the time in black silk pyjamas looking seductive,' I replied. 'But, a man wants to feel loved; wants to feel that he is desired; wants to feel 'a man'. And that is done not only in the bedroom but all the time, by building him up; by making him important to the children – not sniggering at him and running him down – by praising him to his friends; and by flattering him to his face.'

'I see what you mean,' Tana said. 'One forgets to praise one's own husband.'

'It's so easy to get into the habit of bickering in a marriage,' I said. 'It's difficult to keep the desire and excite-

118

ment alive. And, yet, after all, that is a woman's job. Men are too tired and, most of them, too poor, nowadays, to keep a wife and a mistress. But perhaps, in some cases, the competition of a mistress might wake up some of those bored, cheating wives, who don't make their home a place of comfort and security and who treat their husbands as though they were extra servants coming home in the evening to help with the washing-up.'

'Making them wear plastic aprons!' Tana muttered.

'A plastic apron is enough to make any man impotent!' I stormed. 'Women who put one on a man deserve all they get, and what they get is a man who is too indifferent to make love to them because they, themselves, are no longer desirable. So, they get old, frustrated, withered and ugly!'

CHAPTER X

Plan for Youth

'Please let me start on your Youth Plan,' Tana pleaded.
'Is that what you call it?' I laughed.

'Of course,' she replied, 'and you refused to let me buy
the things I wanted until I understood why I needed
them, but now I intend to take off!'

'Very well,' I replied. 'I will tell you what I think will
keep you as attractive and gay as you look today.'

'At fifty?' Tana moaned.

'A woman is as old as she looks,' I quoted. 'So, here is
my Plan for you to remain looking a very young forty-
five for at least the next fifteen years!'

'And what happens after that?' Tana enquired.

'We shall, I hope, have got much more knowledgeable
about how to live young,' I replied.

'And how shall I know about these new discoveries?'
Tana asked.

'Read a clever monthly magazine called *'Here's
Health'*,' I replied. 'It costs only 1/6d., but there's
nothing that happens as regards natural health that you
won't find reported in it and discussed.'

'Good! That's one question out of the way,' Tana exclaimed. 'Now, start on the plan.'

'One moment!' I said. 'Let me repeat one thing which
must never be forgotten. You must eat the right things.
It is no use destroying your body with bad food and
then expecting vitamins to make you young and beauti-

ful. Most people today eat three meals a day and are under-nourished. You must stick to the rules of plenty of protein, no white sugar, no starch, no milk; and do remember that your Health Store is your greatest friend.'

'They are hard to find,' Tana protested.

'Not any more,' I replied. 'The wave of health consciousness sweeping this country and America means that Health Stores are springing up like mushrooms. Already in England we have nearly one thousand and in one month I performed the opening ceremony of two more.'

'But, bully your butcher to provide you with what they call 'traditionally fed' meat – that means without chemicals – and do try and grow a few vegetables yourself. Even the tiniest garden will produce valuable, compost grown green-stuff and I have a friend who grows lettuces and tomatoes in window-boxes and mustard-and-cress on flannel.'

'Vitamin C,' Tana murmured.

'Exactly! And wonderful for your looks,' I smiled. 'And now, here is the next part of the Youth Plan.'

I handed Tana a piece of paper on which I had written: 'Take every day:

2 Gev-E-Tabs
4 Bone Meal
6 Healthcrafts Vitamin E Compleat
4 Healthcrafts Vitamin A Compleat
4 Healthcrafts Vitamin B Compleat
4 Acerola (Vitamin C)

121

\+ Bio-Strath
\+ Celaton or Celaton CH3 Plus.'

'Celaton!' Tana exclaimed. 'That's something new! What is it?'

'It is an amazing scientific rejuvenator,' I replied. 'The tablets contain all the bio-chemical substances which are necessary to keep our cells well and active. I cannot tell you how wonderful Celaton is, not only for people like yourself, who want to remain looking and feeling young, but for the really old, ill and convalescent. I gave Celaton to a woman on the verge of a nervous breakdown and she has thanked me over and over again for saving her sanity. In sexual troubles; for gastric and duodenal ulcers; for bronchitis; sinus infections; Asthma; and even the initial stages of multiple sclerosis, Celaton is like a miracle!'

'It sounds fantastic!' Tana exclaimed.

'It is,' I answered. 'And, for you, it is how to put back the clock. I recommended Celaton tablets to a woman of seventy-two, who actually looked older and was definitely slowing down mentally as well as physically. In a few weeks her face had lost its lines and her skin glowed with good health. She was happy and energetic and told me everyone asked her if she had been for a holiday.'

'I must take Celaton!' Tana said solemnly.

'Two in the morning and two in the evening, before meals,' I said. 'There are two sorts of tablets – the ordinary ones and the Special Tablets, which are much stronger. There are also two sorts of Celaton CH3 tablets one gives tremendous energy the other labelled Plus is for sex.'

122

'Which am I to buy?' Tana asked.

'At fifty, I should take the special Tablets,' I replied, 'either of Celaton or Celaton CH3 Plus.'

'Now, tell me what I should use on my face,' Tana said.

'One thing you mustn't do is to use the same cream indefinitely,' I replied. 'When my children were young they had eczema and I found that every new ointment appeared to disperse the eczema miraculously. 'We've discovered the cure!' I used to cry, and then, after a few days, back came the eczema. This taught me that our skin reacts excitedly, like us, to something new; then it needs change.'

'So don't buy large pots!' Tana said.

'The smallest possible!' I agreed. 'Creams, like food, should always be fresh; and do throw away the last dregs if you stop using them. They are often as bad for the skin as old medicines – which have stood in the cupboard for years – are bad for your body.'

'Small amounts!' Tana said. 'But, of what?'

'I'm going to make you a chart,' I replied. 'And do remember that I only recommend what I have tried myself. There must be many excellent creams which I haven't yet met and there are also some people who won't benefit by what suits me. Keep an open mind on cosmetics and be inquisitive about new products. At the same time, don't be deceived by pretty packaging and fullsome advertisements. Look at the ingredients and, most important of all, make quite certain they are pure, of herbal and vegetable extraction and free of chemicals. Beauty Without Cruelty publishes a brochure which contains a list of all the cosmetics made without animal ingredients – which are bad for the skin.'

'I must get that,' Tana cried.

'Write to Beauty Without Cruelty, 49 Upper Montagu Street, London. W.1,' I told her. 'The organisation was started by a dear friend of mine, Lady Dowding, wife of the famous Air Marshal. It is a non-profit-making concern which fights the terrible cruelty inflicted on animals by some cosmetic manufacturers. Their own preparations are marvellous and contain vital properties from fruit, flowers, nut and plant oils. Lady Dowding told me that her Flowers of Lilac Cream is scented with real lilacs and the Rose Petal Nights Cream with real roses!'

'It sounds too glamorous for words,' Tana enthused.

'It is,' I replied, 'and I will put some of their preparations down on my chart but they have lots more you ought to try.

CHART FOR BEAUTY FOR THE OVER FORTIES

(Prices and addresses at back of book)

The Face. First thing on waking, smooth Celaton Moisture Cream on your face; leave as long as possible.

Use Cyclax Contour Film to tighten the skin; let it dry.

If you are living or working in a city or town, use Cyclax Glam-o-tint – it gives your face a glow.

Or Beauty Without Cruelty Myrrh Foundation Cream. Or Biokosma's Liquid Foundation.

If you are living in or visiting the country, use Elizabeth Arden Sunproof Cream as a foundation.

It protects and heals the skin. Rough weather is *not* good for the skin, so keep it covered, and I find Sunproof Cream is the best protection I know.

Powder with Cyclax Face Powder. This is pure and when you have made up with it you can go all day and all the evening without repowdering. I always recommend it for working girls.

Lipstick. Be careful how you choose a lipstick. There are six dyes used in lipstick in this country which have been banned for three years in the U.S.A. as cancer inducing. Read Beauty Without Cruelty list for safety.

Eyeshadow and Eyeliner. Use Eyelure. Also, their false eyelashes – they are the best in the world. My daughter and I use Meltonian Shoe Cream on our eyelashes instead of mascara. This prevents them from breaking, but it must be removed at night with cold cream. I use the same Queen Products Cold Cream with which I cream my face on pieces of cheap gauze.

Night Time. First cleanse with Queen Products Cold Cream. This is absolutely pure, very cheap and effective. It is a mistake to use the same nourishing cream for too long. First try Celaton's Night Star for a month. It is marvellously smooth and leaves the skin especially refined and free of all blemishes. Then go on to Zodiac's Face Conditioning Cream. This is particularly good for dry ageing skins, and is also an anti-wrinkle moisturiser. This cream also works miracles on a crepey neck.

As a change from these I have tried and can recommend:
Biokosma's Pure Skin Food and lovely soft Vanishing
Cream.
Winston's Placenta Cream with Wheat Germ Oil.
Beauty Without Cruelty's Avocado Satin Cream – pure
and delicious.
New Era's Hymosa, smooth and lovely, which contains
the potentized Biochemic Tissue Salts.
Maria Hornés' Ego-syl – excellent when your skin is
dry or the weather is very cold.
For skins that have already aged, after illness, 'flu, and
certainly twice a week, use the marvellous new enzyme
cream Night Star Special. This is expensive but after
many years of research it claims new skins for old.
Wrinkles come from lack of elasticity because the skin
ages and cell debris lies round the surface. Night Star
Special cream removes the old, expended skin cells and
stimulates new, healthy ones to replace them. It is the
most wonderful rejuvenating cream I have ever found.
I can see my lines softening and beginning to disappear.

Neck. Cyclax Neo Juven and Zodiac Creams are the
best neck rejuvenators I know. After two or three nights
you can see the difference.

Teeth. Sarakan Toothpaste, from the toothbrush tree –
makes the gums both look and feel healthy
or
Inter-Medic's Pardontex Toothpaste and brush –
strengthens the gums and the brush really cleans.
At the Cancer Victims and Friends Convention in Los
Angeles it was reported that a doctor found fluorides in

126

the tissues of 156 cancer patients and that 121 of these had not been drinking fluoridated water. But, on checking, it was found they had all used fluoridated tooth paste.

Hair. Never brush your hair if it is inclined to be thin. Wash with Rosemary Shampoo by Culpeper, or, Lotus Flowers from Beauty Without Cruelty, or, Plant Oil Shampoo by Charles Perry, or, China Balm Cream Shampoo by Cathay of Bournemouth.

Hands. A placenta cream is much better than any hand cream and does remove wrinkles. I use Celaton Placenta Cream, or Winston's.

Bath. Zodiac's Bath Treatment, stimulating and good for the skin.
Winston's Bain Bleu Foam Bath.
Creighton's Forest Flowers.
Finnish Pine Bath.
Charles Perry Seaweed Bath Essence (cheap and good).
Tidman's Bath Sea Salt.
For glambrous evenings:
Estée Lauder's Youth Dew Oil.
Floris' Stephanotis Bath Oil.

Body. Use Creighton's Body Lotion.
Soap. I don't advise soap on the face but if you must wash with it use Hymosa. It is a really pure soap

for delicate skins. I also use Culpeper's Green Lettuce, Malmaison, Stephanotis soaps, and Alfonal's C.N.S. – Completely Natural Soap (unscented).

'Is that all?' Tana asked.

'What more do you want?' I asked. 'Try to use a little of what is pure and good, not a lot of what is rubbish. In the same way, buy a small pot of an · expensive nourishing cream from one of the firms I have mentioned rather than a cheap, large pot which, as often as not, is full of dangerous chemicals or animal extracts which can damage your skin.'

'Never use cheap face powder. Never buy a lipstick made by an unknown firm. Remember, always, that substances are absorbed by the skin and can harm other parts of the body.'

'I never thought of that,' Tana said. 'I will be careful but I'm so excited to think what a difference all you have told me will make to my looks.'

'Hope and happiness are great beautifiers,' I smiled, 'and, most of all, love. I have already told you that beauty comes from within.'

'I know, from the stomach!' Tana laughed.

'Yes, of course, but also from the heart,' I replied. 'Give to those you meet; not only your money – any fool with a bank balance can do that – but your heart. It is the warmth, the sympathy, the compassion and the love we give to others which make us, as women, really fulfil our destiny.'

'And what is that?' Tana asked.

'To leave,' I replied, 'the world a lovelier place because we have passed through it.'

NATURAL VITAMINS FOR THE OVER FORTIES

A deficiency of these vitamins may be accompanied by the symptoms listed, but if these symptoms persist it is best to consult your doctor or The Van Straten Clinic, 6 De Walden Street, London W.1.
FOUNDATION VITAMIN: GEV-E-TABS.

VITAMIN A
Deficiency can cause
Sensitivity to bright light; lesions of the skin; rough, dry skin; inability to store fat; lowered resistance to infections; sinus; poor development of teeth, bones; hastens senility, reduces life span.
Present in Healthcrafts Vitamin A Compleat and their Super 'A' (25,000 i.u.), 'Sustain A' (25,000 i.u.), 'Super Halibut Liver Oil', 'Super Cod Liver Oil'.

Vitamin A, the 'Anti-Infection Vitamin, helps maintain health of eyes, nose, throat, mouth and skin. Essential to the production and support of healthy bone cells and male virility. Without Vitamin A, vision in low light becomes seriously impaired.

VITAMIN B.I. THIAMIN
Deficiency can cause
Loss of appetite; mental depression and nervous upsets;

fatigue; headaches; loss of muscle tone; loss of memory; hyper-sensitivity to noise; insomnia; diarrhoea; oedema to the legs.

Present in

'Super B.I.' (25 mg.), 'Sustain B.I.' (25 mg.), 'Liver-Plus', 'Super Brewer's Yeast'. Healthcrafts B Compleat.

Vitamin B.I., the 'Anti-Fatigue Vitamin', helps prevent nervous conditions and depression. A unique link in metabolism, it is responsible for the release of energy.

VITAMIN B.2. RIBOFLAVIN

Deficiency can cause

Digestive disturbances; poor appetite; cracked and sore lips; forms of dermatitis; dryness of skin; loss of hair; eyesight degeneration.

Present in

'Super B2' (10 mg.), 'Sustain B2' (10 mg.). Healthcrafts B Compleat.

Vitamin B.2 is essential for the complete utilisation of protein and, like all vitamins of the 'B' Complex, is concerned with the health of the skin and nerves. It is prescribed for mouth sores and is beneficial to the eyes.

VITAMIN B.6. PYRIDOXINE

Deficiency can cause

Skin disorders; anaemia; irritability; bad muscle tone; eczema.

Present in

'Super B.6.' (10 mg.), 'Sustain B6' (10 mg.), 'Anti-sat', Healthcrafts B Compleat.

Vitamin B.6. is particularly recognised for the prevention and treatment of skin complaints and is employed in the metabolism of fat and protein. As part of the 'B' Complex it shares responsibility for the health of the nerves and assists other vitamins to safeguard heart, intestines and muscles.

VITAMIN B.12
Deficiency can cause
Poor appetite and growth in children; anaemia with tiredness and poor appetite; lack of muscular co-ordination.
Present in
'Super B.12' (25 mcg.), 'Sustain B.12' (25 mcg.), Healthcrafts B Compleat.

Vitamin B.12 is essential for the formation of red blood cells and is particularly important to the nervous system. It has excellent tonic properties and is a nutritional 'must' where meat consumption is low. Vegetarians, in particular, are all too often deficient in Vitamin B.12. Surveys show also that many older people have low blood levels of B.12.

VITAMIN C
Deficiency can cause
Scurvy; bleeding gums; fatigue; vulnerability to catching colds, sinus infection; lowered resistance to disease; general lowering of health; apathy.
Present in
'Acerola' tablets (delicious to suck), 'Vita-Mine' Syrup Rose Hip tablets, 'Super C' (200 mg.), 'Sustain C' (200 mg.), 'Bio-Flavons', Healthcrafts C Compleat.

Vitamin C affords general protection and is prescribed for the prevention and treatment of colds, 'flu, etc. Vitamin C replacement is required daily.

VITAMIN D
Deficiency can cause
Lowered calcium and phosphorus content of the blood; defective calcification in bones; poor teeth; rickets in children; osteomalacia in adults.
Present in
'Super Halibut Liver Oil', 'Super Cod Liver Oil', 'Vegetarian Bone Meal', 'Super Bone Meal'.

Vitamin D is essential to the young for the growth of healthy bones, teeth, etc. It is equally important during later years when it is needed for the maintenance and renewal of bone tissue. Vitamin D also protects against muscular weakness and fatigue.

VITAMIN E
Deficiency can cause
Menopause problems; increased senility; loss of sexual vigour; sterility; muscular and cardiovascular difficulties; circulatory disorders; inability to utilise other vitamins; varicose veins.
Present in
'Super Wheat Germ Oil', 'Super E' (100 i.u.), 'Sustain E' (100 i.u.), Healthcrafts E Compleat.

Vitamin E, known as the 'Vitality Vitamin', is believed to oxygenate the tissues, reducing the fat content of the blood and assisting in the utilisation of carbohydrates and proteins, the main constituents of food. Vitamin E is also essential for the metabolism of unsaturated fatty acids. It is also the 'Youth and Sex Vitamin'.

VITAMIN F
Deficiency can cause
High cholesterol; fragile artery walls; high blood pressure; aching legs.
Present in
'Super Lecithin', 'Anti-Sat'.

IODINE
Deficiency can cause
Retarded growth; enlarged thyroid glands (goitre); lowered metabolism; mental and physical sluggishness; lack of energy.
Present in
'Super Kelp'.

MAGNESIUM
Deficiency can cause
Brittle bones; taut nerves; lowered calcium; muscular weakness and fatigue.
Present in
'Dolomite', 'Bone Meal'.

ZINC
Deficiency can cause
Impaired growth.
Present in
'Super Kelp'.

ADD TO THESE
BIO-STRATH – the amazing Health Elixir.
CELATON CH3 – regenerates and recreates dying cells.
FLORODIX – the perpetual digestible iron toxic.

MAGIC SLIMMING DIET*

Magic menu

1. Breakfast $\frac{1}{2}$ GRAPEFRUIT or unsweetened GRAPE-
FRUIT JUICE, 2 EGGS and 2 slices of BA-
CON, minimum (you may eat 12 slices of
BACON and 12 EGGS, any style, if you
want) weak TEA, NO CREAM, NO SUGAR.

2. Lunch $\frac{1}{2}$ GRAPEFRUIT, MEAT, any style, any
amount with a SALAD, as much as you can
eat with any dressing that contains no
SUGAR, – glass of water.

3. Dinner $\frac{1}{2}$ GRAPEFRUIT, MEAT, any style, any
amount with gravy providing that is has
not been thickened with FLOUR. Of course,
you may substitute FISH for MEAT. Any
GREEN – YELLOW, or RED VEGETA-
BLES, as much as you can eat, and SALAD
as above.

4. Bedtime Fresh TOMATO JUICE, SKIMMED MILK
snack POWDER, or MOLAT.

At each meal you must eat until you are full, until you
cannot possibly eat more.

* Based on a diet from a Clinic in the U.S.A.

134

Don't eliminate anything: for example don't skip BACON at breakfast or omit SALAD at dinner. It is this combination of food that burns up accumulated fat.

The GRAPEFRUIT is important because it acts as a CATALYST that starts the fat-burning process.

No COFFEE – it is thought to affect the INSULIN balance that hinders burning-up processes.

No eating between meals. If you can eat the combination of foods suggested until you are stuffed, you won't be hungry between meals.

Note that this diet COMPLETELY ELIMINATES SUGARS AND STARCHES which form LIPOIDS and LIPOIDS are what forms fat.

You can lose 10 lbs. in ten days. There will be no weight loss the first 4 days but you will suddenly drop 5 lbs. on the 5th day. Thereafter you lose 1 lb. a day until the 10th day. Then you will lose 1-½ lbs. every 2 days until you get down to your proper weight.

DIET FOR 14 DAYS ONLY. REST A MONTH. REPEAT ONLY IF NECESSARY.

NOTE: It is very important to take 4 Bone Meal tablets every day to avoid the citrus acid of the grapefruit damaging the teeth.

MOLAT is a basic dietary food from powdered vitamin oil, milk protein and wheat germ extract, obtainable from:–
Biocosmetics (London) Ltd. 128 High Street, Edgware, Middx.

Here is a list of cures for specific complaints

ACNE	CELATON'S SPECIAL ACNE TREATMENT.
ASTHMA	KNOWLES BREATHING COURSE, wich is marvellous with POTTERS ASTHMA AND BRONCHITIS HERBS, plus vitamins E and A. Take 2 Gev–E–Tabs, 8 vitamin E, 4 vitamin A, 4 Bone Meal, plus Bio-Strath No. 12.
BLOOD PRESSURE – High	RUTIN–'T' and RUTIVITE TABLETS.
CATARRH	NEW ERA COMBINATION 'J', or, BENHOMICS TREATMENT plus 1 Gev–E–Tabs, 3 vitamin A, 4 Acerola, 4 Bone Meal, Bio-Strath No. 12. Forbidden – Milk; starchy foods white bread.
CHILBLAINS	NEW ERA COMBINATION 'P', plus 4 Bone Meal, 2 Gev–E–Tabs, 4 Acerola a day. Plus LUSTY'S CHILBLAIN OINTMENT.
CIRCULATION – Poor	6 vitamin E plus 2 Gev–E–Tabs, plus BIO-STRATH CIRCULATION FORMULA No. 1.
CLINIC	THE VAN STRATEN CLINIC at 6 De Walden St., off Wimpole Street, London W. 1. has every

treatment under one roof – Naturopathy, Osteopathy, Acupuncture, Homoeopathy, Iri-dology and Electro-Therapy. Do consult the Director,
Mr. Michael Van Straten, N.D., D.O., M.B.N.O.A., Dip. Ac., M. Ac. A.

COLDS AND INFLUENZA	CULPEPER'S INFLUENZA MIXTURE. This is a wonderful mixture which really does clear up a cold and cure influenza. I always take it very hot with a tablespoonful of honey and it is delicious. Increase usual vitamin intake.
COMPLEXION – Bad or sallow	CULPEPER'S BEAUTY PILLS, plus 1 Gev–E–Tabs, 2 vitamin A, 4 vitamin B6, 4 Bone Meal, Bio-Strath Elixir.
CONSTIPATION	CULPEPER'S APERIENT TEA; or HEALTHCRAFTS' INNER FRESH; or POTTER'S SENNA POD TABLETS; or BIO-VAX SUPPOSITORIES. These should be used by anyone with a delicate digestion.
CYSTITIS	BIO - STRATH KIDNEY - BLADDER FORMULA No. 7; or CULPEPER'S COUCH GRASS HERB TEA; or BENHOMIC TREAT-

137

MENT FOR CYSTITIS.
Increase usual vitamin intake.
Note: Middle-aged women who do not wear wollen pants during the winter months are asking for trouble.

DANDRUFF	4 SUPER VITAMIN A plus 2 Gev–E–Tabs, 4 Bone Meal, and Bio-Strath Elixir daily.
DIGESTIVE AND INTESTINAL TROUBLE	HEALTHCRAFTS' FLORUS – the only form of Acidophilus which can survive in the human intestine.
FACE MASKS	DR. GRANDEL'S FERMENT SKIN MASK, made from herbal extracts. Excellent for large pores, pimply, greasy skins and for blackheads. Or, CHARLES PERRY'S WHEAT GERM AND YEAST BEAUTY MASK.
FATIGUE	This invariably comes from wrong feeding. See that your diet has plenty of protein, i.e. meat, fish, eggs, end plenty of vitamins, plus 3 Brewers' Yeast after each meal, 2 Gev–E–Tabs, 4 Bone Meal, and Bio-Strath Elixir. And add VIT-AMINO HI-PROTEIN BEVERAGE – this contains 18 essential Animo-Acids besides Wheat Germ and other

138

proteins. On the tin it says 'mix with warm milk'. Skimmed milk powder is best – use Snow Queen. Or, I prefer warm blackcurrant juice to which I add a spoonful of honey. When mixed together it is delicious.

LIVER-PLUS is another great source of energy and easy to take around in your pocket – take 3 after each meal. CELETON also prevents fatigue and rejuvenates.

FEET – Tired or Swollen

CELATON'S KUMFOOT. Take 4 Lecithin, 4 vitamin E, 1 Gev-E-tab, 4 Bone Meal daily.

FIBROSITIS

Impulsator treatment from THE VAN STRATEN CLINIC, 6 De Walden Street, London W.I. or NEW ERA COMBINATION 'I'; or BIO-STRATH RHEUM-ELEXIR No. 5; plus 2 Gev–E–Tabs, 6 Super Vitamin E, 2 vitamin A, 6 Bone Meal, 4 Acerola, 4 Brewers' Yeast.

HAIR – Dry, greasy, falling out.

Your hair is a barometer of your health. First take vitamins, especially vitamin B.2. Bio Strath helps hair to grow. So does vitamin E (minimum dose 4 capsules a day). Use shampoos without chemicals or detergents.

For Premature
greyness.

HAYFEVER

HEART TROUBLE
(Also Fatigue, Liver
Complaints, Circula-
latory trouble, Blood
Pressure, Palpitation)

Beauty without Cruelty and Cul-
peper's shampoos are excellent.
For very dry hair CHARLES PER-
RY'S WILD HONEY SHAMPOO
rinse, use PLANT OILSHAMPOO,
leave for 2 minutes and rinse.
For very bad dandruf use DAN-
NEX EUCALYPTOL SHAMPOO
and also use their treatment.
HEATH AND HEATHER EX-
TRACT or ROSEMARY AND BIO-
STRATH ELIXIR.
RAYNER & PENNYCOOK'S COM-
FREY TABLETS; plus 1 Gev-
E-Tab, 4 Vitamin A, 4 Acerola,
4 Bone Meal, Bio- Strath Elixir.
There is an amazing new injec-
tion from Hungary called EM-
BRYCORDIN. This is the extract
from a pure embryonal heart. At
first, Embrycordin was used
only for heart diseases especially
in the aged. Then the immediate
difference it made to the general
health of the patient persuaded
the doctors in the Clinic to use it
on every patient whatever the
disease for which they were ad-
mitted. The results were fantastic; patients felt better, looked
better, were younger and more

active. I have suffered for years from a low blood pressure and tried hundreds of cures; only Embrycordin has raised it to normal.

HERBS

There are HERBS for every ailment, every disease – this is Nature's remedy. The oldest Herbalist in this Country and the most famous is CULPEPER, 21 Bruton Street, London W.1. I advise everyone interested in natural health to send for their Catalogue (1/6d.) and price lists. Herbs are cheap, but used intelligently they have an amazing effect on the body, mind and face. For books on Herbs read 'Green Medicine' and 'Hearts Ease' by Mrs. Leyel from Culpeper.

INVALIDS

JECOROL is a natural vitamin preparation with Calcium Salts. It builds the patient up and I recommend it for growing children and nursing mothers besides the usual vitamins.

MENOPAUSE

VITAMIN E is essential and I advise 6 capsules a day, plus BIO-STRATH FEMINAL FORMULA No. 10 or HEALTCRAFTS' GOLDEN SEAL. Increase all vitamins, especially Bone Meal.

MIGRAINE	ELECTRIC ACUPUNCTURE from The Clinic, 6 De Walden Street, London W.1., plus 1 Gev-E-Tab, 4 vitamin E; plus lots of Honey, Bio-Strath Elixir and Celaton Tablets. Forbidden – coffee, chocolate, tea, oranges, milk.
MOUTH ULCERS	STANNOXYL. Mouth ulcers are usually caused by a vitamin deficiency. Take 1 Gev–E–Tab, 4 Bone Meal, 2 Acerola, plus Bio-Strath Elixir.
NECK – Wrinkled and Crepey	CYCLAX'S NECKLINE in the daytime. CYCLAX'S NEO JUVEN Cream at night.
OBESITY	BIO-STRATH SLIMMING FORMULA No. 11; slow, safe, but doesn't slim everybody. Or, CELATON SPECIAL SLIMMING TABLETS; safe; takes away the appetite and must be taken with Celaton Tablets. No-one should slim without taking vitamins. 2 Gev–E–Tabs, 4 Bone Meal Tablets a day will be sufficient for most young people. For those over forty-five, Bio-Strath Elixir as well is most important and prevents premature ageing.

See also 'Magic Slimmimg Diet' page 191A.

PEPTIC ULCER	DE-NOL. A fantastic cure from South Africa. Patients are able to eat a full diet within 3 days of starting the treatment.
PERIOD PAINS	BIO-STRATH FEMINAL FORMULA No. 10. Golden Seal. Eat no fruit three days before and during the period. Increase vitamins.
PILES	CULPEPER'S PILE HERBS; or PREPARATION H; or POTTER'S PILE MIXTURE in bottle. Daily, 2 Gev–E–Tab, 6 Super vitamin E, 4 Acerola. Forbidden – coffee, alcohol, citrus fruits.
RHEUMATISM	BIO-STRATH RHEUM-ELIXIR No. 5; plus 2 Gev–E–Tabs, 6 to 10 Super vitamin E, 4 B.12, 4 vitamin A, 2 Halibut Oil capsules, 4 Bone Meal, 4 Acerola, 3 Super Brewers' Yeast after every meal. Or, BENHOMIC TREATMENT FOR RHEUMATISM; Or, LUSTY'S RHEUMATISM HERBS. Both with vitamins and CULPEPER'S RHEUMATISM HERB TEA.
SMOKING	'STOP SMOKING COURSE' from

	APOTHECARY CATHAY. This works with some people; you need willpower as well. Bio-Strath Elixir helps to stop the craving.
SPOTS	SPOTOWAY.
STYES	STANNOXYL.
TUMMY – Fat	Use MARIA HORNÉS' BOBAL – which is a rubber ball on a flexible handle. A friend of mine took two inches off her tummy and hips while watching television.
VITALITY – Lack of	GINSENG (ARALIA QUINQUEFOLIA)

This is a root known from the most ancient times in China and is the most famous medicinal herb in the world for adult vitality. The Chinese believe it gives them sexual virility but it is also one of the best and safest remedies for mental and nervous exhaustion. Only imported root of the highest possible quality is used by CATHAY OF BOURNE-MOUTH. But it is a very expensive herb that few can afford.

VER-O-ZEST. A lift-you-up tonic for the hard up. Contains six marvellous herbs. A friend told me he found it 'as good as a glass of champagne.'

VEINS (BROKEN) La Jeunesse special cream.

WARTS CULPEPER'S CORN AND WART PAINT – slow but sure. Or, LUSTY'S CORN AND WART OINTMENT.

WRINKLES I know of nothing better than Night Star Special. This amazing enzyme cream really does rejuvenate the whole face and makes the skin youthful, clean, pure and unblemished. It's sensational on crepey eyelids, thinning necks and the backs of ageing hands. Take 6 Healthcrafts Vitamin E at the same time, 4 tablets of Celaton CH3 Plus and Biocosmetics Whole Wheat Germ Tablets. In a week you'll see an unbelievable difference.

STOP PRESS

SEXUAL TROUBLES CH3 which is the amazing combination of H3 and Celaton Biostimulin produces a resurgence of sexual interest and vitality. Also prevents premature ageing, insomnia, depression, gastric and duodenal complaints.

145

Addresses and Prices of Products Mentioned in the Youth Secret

A
ACEROLA – Alfonal
Health Stores   56p
ACNE Treatment
Biocosmetics
128 High Street,
Edgware, Middx.   £1·00
ACUPUNCTURE Electric
The Clinic,
J De Walden Street,
London W.1.
ALGEMARIN Seaweed Bath Elixir
Vitality Fare,
5 Thayer Street,
London W.1.
AMPLEX
Any Chemist
ANTI-SAT – Alfonal
Health Stores   32 days   46p

B
BIOKOSMA
Health Stores or
Inter-Medics Ltd.,
Commerce Lane,
Letchworth, Herts.

Nourishing Cream	**61p**
Vanishing Cream	**61p**
Face Lotion	**75p**

BEAUTY WITHOUT CRUELTY
Health Stores and
49 Upper Montagu Street,
London W.1.

Rose Petal Night Cream	**44p**
Flowers of Lilac Cream	**34p**
Myrrh Foundation Cream	**52½p**
Avocado Satin Cream	**£1·07½**
Lotus Flowers Shampoo	**39p**

BENHOMICS
Miller Street,
Radcliffe, Lancs.

Treatment for Rheumatism	**37½p**
Treatment for Catarrh	**37½p**

BIO-STRATH – Stratenport
Health Stores

Elixir	**£1·35**
Rheum-Elixir No. 5	**£1·50**
Kidney-Bladder Formulo No. 7	**£1·50**
Feminal Formula No. 10	**£1·50**
Slimming Formula No. 11	**£1·50**
Chest Formula No. 12	**£1·50**

BIO-VAX Suppositories
Health Stores   **10 for 62½p**

BOBAL – Maria Hornes
16 Davies Street,
London W.1.   **£1·05**

BONE MEAL – Alfonal
Health Stores   500 for 52½p
BREWERS' YEAST – Alfonal
Health Stores   250 for 19p

C
CATHAY OF BOURNEMOUTH
124 Christchurch Road,
Bournemouth
  'Stop Smoking Course'   **£1·00**
  'Ginseng'   **100 tablets £2·25**
CHARLES PERRY
Health Stores or
155 Pitshanger Lane,
Ealing, London W.5.
  Wild Honey Shampoo   **29½p**
  Plant Oil Shampoo
  Seaweed Bath Essence   **27½p**
CELATON
Health Stores or
Biocosmetics,
128 High Street,
Edgware, Middx.
  Celaton Tablets   **1 month's supply £2·00**
  Special Strength Slimming Tablets   **£3·00**
  Night Star   **£2·90**
  Moisture Cream   **£2·20**
  Face Lift   **£1·77½**
  Placenta Oil   **£3·00**
  Night Star Special   **£5·00**

Kumfoot 52½p
Celaton CH3 Plus for Sex £3·00
Celaton CH3 for Energy £2·90

CHILBLAIN Ointment – Lusty's
Health Stores 15p

COMFREY Tablets for Hay Fever – *Rayner and*
Pennycook,
Covett Avenue,
Shepperton, Middx. 150 for 32p

C.N.S. Completely Natural Soap – Alfonal
Health Stores 6½p

CREIGHTON
Health Stores or
Water Lane,
Storrington,
Sussex.
Forest Flowers Bath Oil 27½p
Body Lotion 36p

CULPEPER
Health Stores or,
21 Bruton Street,
London W.1.
Aperient Tea 4 ozs. 19p
Beauty Pills 24½p
Elder Flowers Cream 29½p
Foundation Cream 48p
Milk of Lilies Cleansing Lotion 25p
Mountain Water 37p
Rosemary Shampoo 19p
Slim Tablets 24½p

Soaps – various	from 14p
Corn and Wart Paint	25p
Pile Herbs	15½p

CYCLAX
65 South Molton Street,
London W.1.

Face Powder	46p
Neo Juven	£2·12½
Contorfilm	£1·08
Neckline	59p
GlamOtint	46p

D

DANNEX Eucalyptol Shampoo – Alfonal

Health Stores	52½p
Eucalyptol Treatment	32½p

DE-NOL –   a bottle £4·50
Peptinol Ltd.
80 Elswick Road,
Newcastle-upon-Tyne 4. or
Boots Cash Chemists,
Piccadilly Circus,
London W.1.

DOLOMITE – Alfonal

Health Stores	100 tablets 34p

E

EGO–SYL – Maria Hornés
16 Davies Street,
London W.1.   £1·10

EMBRYCORDIN
Biocosmetics,
128 High Street,
Edgware, Middx.   **10 injections £2·00**
EYES: Shadow and False Eyelashes – Eyelure
Salon: Let's Face It,
8 Grosvenor Street, London W.1.   **Shadowmatt 27½p**

F
FLORUS – Alfonal
Health Stores   **90p**
FINNISH Pine Bath – Alfonal
Health Stores   **a bottle 24½p**

G
GEV-E-TABS – Alfonal
Health Stores   **16 days 57½p**
GOLDEN SEAL – Alfonal   **3 weeks 50½p**
Health Stores
DR. GRANDEL's Ferment Skin Mask – *Cellular*
Medicaments Ltd.,
136 High Street,
Edgware, Middx.
GINSENG (Aralia Quinquefolia)
See Cathay of Bournemouth.

H
H. 3 Injections and Tablets
The Clinic,
6 De Walden Street, London W.1.

152

HERB Formula D – Alfonal
Health Stores $38\frac{1}{2}$p
HEATH AND HEATHER
Health Stores
   Ver–O–Zest   **43p**
   Ver–O–Vine   **43p**
   Extract of Rosemary
HYMOSA Soap
          Skin Lotion
New Era Lab:
87 Saffron Hill,
London E.C.1.

I
INNER FRESH – Alfonal $20\frac{1}{2}$p
Health Stores or
Meadrow, Godalming,
Surrey. $38\frac{1}{2}$p
INTER-MEDICS
Deanrow, Pasture Road,
Letchworth,
Herts.
   Pardontax Toothpaste and Brush $72\frac{1}{2}$p
   Jecoral $52\frac{1}{2}$p

J
JECORAL – Intermedics
Deanrow, Pasture Road,
Letchworth,
Herts. $52\frac{1}{2}$p

K
KELP Tablets – Alfonal
Health Stores   **250 for 30p**
KNOWLES Method of Breath Training
Ingleby, Cherry Rise,
Kings Road, Chalfont
St. Giles,
Bucks.   **£5·25**
KRETSCHMERS Wheat Germ Cereal – Alfonal
Health Stores   **19p**

L
LECITHIN Tablets – Alfonal
Health Stores   **100 for $26\frac{1}{2}$p**
LIVERPLUS – Alfonal
Health Stores   **100 for 44p**
LUSTY'S
Health Stores or
London Road,
Westcliff-on-Sea,
Essex.
   Rheumatism Herbs $12\frac{1}{2}$p
   Chilblain Ointment $12\frac{1}{2}$p
   Corn and Wart Ointment $12\frac{1}{2}$p

M
MOLAT
Biocosmetics (London) Ltd., $52\frac{1}{2}$p
128 High Street,
Edgware, Middx.

N
NECKLINE – Cyclax
65 South Molton Street,
London W.1. **59p**
NEO JUVEN – Cyclax
65 South Molton Street,
London W.1. **£2·12½**
NEW ERA
87 Saffron Hill, London E.C.1.
    Combination 'I' – Fibrositis **51p**
    Combination 'J' – Catarrh **51p**

P
PEPPERMINT TEA – Heath and Heather
Health Stores **12½p**
PERRY Charles
Health Stores or
155 Pitshanger Lane,
Ealing, London W.5.
    Plant Oil Shampoo **29½p**
    Seaweed Bath Essence **29½p**
    Sunflower Oil **24p**
    Wheat Germ and Yeast Beauty Mask **47½p**
PLACENTA Cream – Celaton
128 High Street
Edgware, Middx.
PLANT OIL SHAMPOO – Charles Perry
Health Stores or
155 Pitshanger Lane,
Ealing, London W.5. **29½p**

POTTERS
Health Stores
    Asthma and Bronchitis Herbs   **12½p**
    Senna Pod Tablets   **12½p**
    Pile Mixture   **27½p**

PREPARATION H
Any Chemist

PUMPKIN SEEDS
Vitality Fare,
5 Thayer Street,
London W.1.   **37½p**

Q

QUEEN PRODUCTS Cold Cream
Boutalls Chemists,
60 Lamb's Conduit Street,
London W.C.1.
    or
Harrods Ltd.,
Knightsbridge,
London S.W.1.

R

ROSE HIP SYRUP: Hip C – Alfonal
Health Stores   **37½p**

RUTIN Products Ltd.
Station Approach,
Wokingham, Berks.
    Rutin 'T'   **1 month's supply 48½p**
    Rutivite Tablets   **48½p**

S

SARAKAN Toothpaste
88 Harley House,
Regents Park,
London N.W.1. 24p

SMOKING (to stop)
Apothecary Cathay,
124 Christchurch Road,
Bournemouth,
Hants. £1·00

SPOTOWAY Acne Treatment
Health Stores or
Pure Plant Products,
8 Hodgson Drive,
Timperley, Cheshire. 29p

STANNOXYL
Any Chemist
SUNPROOF CREAM – Elizabeth Arden 52½p
25 Old Bond Street,
London W.1.

U

ULCERS, Peptic – DE-NOL
Peptinol (G.B.) Ltd.,
80 Elswick Road,
Newcastle-upon-Tyne 4. £4·50

V

VER–O–VINE – Heath and Heather
Health Stores 43p

VER–O–ZEST – Heath and Heather
Health Stores   **43p**
VITAMIN A Super – Alfonal
Health Stores   **92½p**
  Healthcrafts A Compleat   **97½p**
  Healthcrafts B Compleat   **44p**
  Healthcrafts B1   **64p**
  Healthcrafts B2   **52½p**
  Healthcrafts B6   **77½p**
  Healthcrafts B12   **62½p**
  Healthcrafts C – Acerola   **56p**
  Healthcrafts E Super   **£1·06**
  Healthcrafts E Compleat   **£1·12½**
VIT–AMINO Protein Beverage
Health Stores   **1 month's supply £1·25**

W
WHEAT GERM cereal Kretschners – Alfonal
Health Stores   **19p**
W.5 – Milesdon Ltd.
(Dept. HL/12),
11 Queen's Road,
Horsham, Surrey.
WHOLE WHEAT GERM   **£1·30**
Health Stores or
Biocosmetics,
128 High Street,
Edgware, Middx.

Love, Life and Sex

'I've come to say goodbye!' Tana said, looking very glamorous in a coral dress and coat and a jaunty little hat trimmed with quills.

'Goodbye?' I questioned. 'Where are you going?'

'On a second honeymoon,' Tana answered, her eyes sparkling. 'Yes, Barbara, I've been trying out all you told me this last month and, darling, it works!'

'You mean John?' I asked.

'John has been fed, flattered, complimented and cossetted,' Tana answered. 'And, oh dear! I feel I was only just in time to prevent him thinking he was too old for love.'

'He was beginning to think that!' I exclaimed.

'He thought I didn't want him,' Tana explained. 'He was afraid of beginning to make love to me and failing! He was tired because he wasn't eating the right things or having vitamins. What a fool I was!'

'And now?' I asked.

Tana really seemed to blush.

'It's wonderful!' she answered. 'And I think that as we know so much more than we did when we were young, it's better than it ever was!'

'That's right,' I said. 'Love-making should improve with age. I can't say too often that it is an art and an inexhaustible, continual delight.'

'That's what we are both beginning to understand,' Tana

159

agreed. 'And I've remembered that love doesn't like clocks, rules and regulations, conventions or restrictions.'

'Of course it doesn't,' I agreed. 'Only the English think love-making must be in the dark on Saturday night!'

'Well, we're going to Paris for our second honeymoon,' Tana said. 'The French understand a notice on the door saying, 'Do Not Disturb'!'

'Don't forget to have a honeymoon every year,' I told her. 'For many marriages it is the one thing which keeps love alive – a time together away from the house, the children, the business and those interminable telephone calls.'

Tana laughed.

'We are not even telling the office where we are going.'

'Very sensible,' I approved. 'And do remember not to plan your days or do too much. The best time for love-making has always been after lunch, so don't go shopping or to the races – go to bed.'

'We will,' Tana answered, and added: 'Barbara, this is all due to you and I am so grateful.'

'You were a willing and excellent pupil,' I replied. 'And looking at you I know you have found the Youth Secret.'

'It may be love,' Tana smiled. 'But I also need vitamins.'

'Not vitamins but health,' I corrected her. 'It is health which makes life gay, exciting and wonderful – and when there is health there is love and there, in a nutshell, lies the whole Secret of Youth.'